T0259454

Heel Pathology

Guest Editor

GEORGE F. WALLACE, DPM, MBA

CLINICS IN PODIATRIC MEDICINE AND SURGERY

www.podiatric.theclinics.com

Consulting Editor
THOMAS ZGONIS, DPM, FACFAS

July 2010 • Volume 27 • Number 3

SAUNDERS an imprint of ELSEVIER, Inc.

W.B. SAUNDERS COMPANY
A Division of Elsevier Inc.

1600 John F. Kennedy Boulevard • Suite 1800 • Philadelphia, Pennsylvania 19103-2899

http://www.theclinics.com

CLINICS IN PODIATRIC MEDICINE AND SURGERY Volume 27, Number 3
July 2010 ISSN 0891-8422, ISBN-13: 978-1-4377-2487-5

Editor: Patrick Manley

Clinics in Podiatric Medicine and Surgery (ISSN 0891-8422) is published quarterly by Elsevier Inc., 360 Park Avenue South, New York, NY 10010-1710. Months of issue are January, April, July, and October. Business and Editorial Offices: 1600 John F. Kennedy Blvd., Ste. 1800, Philadelphia, PA 19103-2899. Customer Service Office: 3251 Riverport Lane, Maryland Heights, MO 63043. Periodicals postage paid at New York, NY and additional mailing offices. Subscription prices are $252.00 per year for US individuals, $367.00 per year for US institutions, $130.00 per year for US students and residents, $303.00 per year for Canadian individuals, $454.00 for Canadian institutions, $359.00 for international individuals, $454.00 per year for international institutions and $184.00 per year for Canadian and foreign students/residents. To receive student/resident rate, orders must be accompanied by name of affiliated institution, date of term, and the *signature* of program/residency coordinator on institution letterhead. Orders will be billed at individual rate until proof of status is received. Foreign air speed delivery is included in all *Clinics* subscription prices. All prices are subject to change without notice. POSTMASTER: Send address changes to *Clinics in Podiatric Medicine and Surgery*, Elsevier Health Sciences Division, Subscription Customer Service, 3251 Riverport Lane, Maryland Heights, MO 63043. **Customer Service: 1-800-654-2452 (US). From outside of the US, call 314-447-8871. Fax: 314-447-8029. E-mail: JournalsCustomerService-usa@elsevier.com (for print support); JournalsOnlineSupport-usa@elsevier.com (for online support).**

Reprints. For copies of 100 or more of articles in this publication, please contact the Commercial Reprints Department, Elsevier Inc., 360 Park Avenue South, New York, NY 10010-1710. Tel.: 212-633-3812; Fax: 212-462-1935; E-mail: reprints@elsevier.com.

Clinics in Podiatric Medicine and Surgery is covered in *MEDLINE/PubMed (Index Medicus)* and *EMBASE/Excerpta Medica.*

Printed and bound by CPI Group (UK) Ltd, Croydon, CR0 4YY

Transferred to Digital Print 2011

CLINICS IN PODIATRIC MEDICINE AND SURGERY

CONSULTING EDITOR
THOMAS ZGONIS, DPM, FACFAS

Contributors

CONSULTING EDITOR

THOMAS ZGONIS, DPM, FACFAS
Director, Podiatric Surgical Residency and Reconstructive Fellowship Programs;
Chief, Division of Podiatric Medicine and Surgery; Associate Professor, Department
of Orthopedic Surgery, The University of Texas Health Science Center at San Antonio,
San Antonio, Texas

GUEST EDITOR

GEORGE F. WALLACE, DPM, MBA
Director, Podiatry Service; Medical Director, Ambulatory Care Services, University
Hospital, University of Medicine and Dentistry of New Jersey, Newark, New Jersey

AUTHORS

ELIZA ADDIS-THOMAS, DPM
Third Year Resident, Yale-New Haven Hospital, New Haven, Connecticut

RACHEL BALLOCH, DPM, AACFAS
Willimantic, Connecticut

RONALD BELCZYK, DPM
Assistant Professor, Division of Podiatric Medicine and Surgery, Department of
Orthopaedic Surgery, University of Texas Health Science Center at San Antonio,
San Antonio, Texas

KATHERINE CHEN, DPM
Second Year Podiatric Surgical Resident, University Hospital, University of Medicine
and Dentistry of New Jersey, Newark, New Jersey

WARREN A. CHIODO, DPM
Podiatry Resident, Podiatry Service, University Hospital-University of Medicine and
Dentistry of New Jersey, Newark, New Jersey

KEITH D. COOK, DPM, FACFAS
Residency Director, Podiatry Service, University Hospital-University of Medicine and
Dentistry of New Jersey, Newark, New Jersey

SPYRIDON GALANAKOS, MD
Resident, 4th Department of Orthopaedics, KAT General Hospital, Athens, Greece

KEVIN HEALEY, DPM
Diplomate, American Board of Foot and Ankle Surgery, Diplomate,
American Board of Podiatric Orthopedics and Primary Podiatric Medicine,
University of Hospital, University of Medicine and Dentistry of New Jersey, Newark,
New Jersey

GENNADY KOLODENKER, DPM
Podiatric Surgical Resident, University Hospital, University of Medicine and Dentistry
of New Jersey, Newark, New Jersey

ERIC LUI, DPM
Associate, Connecticut Surgical Group, Hartford, Connecticut

GEORGE MACHERAS, MD
Director of Orthopaedic Traumatology, 4th Department of Orthopaedics, KAT General
Hospital, Athens, Greece

ERIN E. MATHEWS, DPM
Second Year Resident, Yale-New Haven Hospital, New Haven, Connecticut

IOANNIS PAPAKOSTAS, MD, PhD
Consultant Orthopaedic Surgeon, General Hospital of Limnos, Limnos, Greece

SONYA L. PEREZ, DPM
Third Year Resident, Yale-New Haven Hospital, New Haven, Connecticut

VASILIOS D. POLYZOIS, MD, PhD
Chief of Orthopaedic Traumatology, 4th Department of Orthopaedics, KAT General
Hospital, Athens, Greece

CRYSTAL L. RAMANUJAM, DPM
Fellow, Postgraduate Research and Clinical Instructor, Division of Podiatric Medicine
and Surgery, Department of Orthopaedic Surgery, University of Texas Health Science
Center at San Antonio, San Antonio, Texas

BRIAN SELBST, DPM
Podiatric Surgical Resident, Division of Podiatric Medicine and Surgery, Department
of Orthopaedic Surgery, University of Texas Health Science Center at San Antonio,
San Antonio, Texas

JOHN J. STAPLETON, DPM
Associate, Foot and Ankle Surgery, VSAS Orthopaedics, Allentown; Clinical Assistant
Professor of Surgery, Penn State College of Medicine, Hershey, Pennsylvania

STEVEN D. VYCE, DPM, FACFAS
Assistant Clinical Professor, Department of Orthopaedics and Rehabilitation, Yale
University School of Medicine, New Haven; Director of Podiatric Medical Education
and Residency Training, Yale/VACT PMS; Chief, Podiatry Section, Veterans Affairs
Connecticut Healthcare Systems, West Haven, Connecticut

JUSTIN WADE, DPM
Podiatric Surgical Resident, Division of Podiatric Medicine and Surgery, Department
of Orthopaedic Surgery, University of Texas Health Science Center at San Antonio,
San Antonio, Texas

GEORGE F. WALLACE, DPM, MBA
Director, Podiatry Service; Medical Director, Ambulatory Care Services, University
Hospital, University of Medicine and Dentistry of New Jersey, Newark, New Jersey

THOMAS ZGONIS, DPM, FACFAS
Director, Podiatric Surgical Residency and Reconstructive Fellowship Programs;
Chief, Division of Podiatric Medicine and Surgery; Associate Professor, Department
of Orthopedic Surgery, The University of Texas Health Science Center at San Antonio,
San Antonio, Texas

Contributors   vi

GEORGE F. WALLACE, DPM, MBA
Director, Podiatry Services, Medical Director, Ambulatory Care Services, University Hospital, University of Medicine and Dentistry of New Jersey, Newark, New Jersey

THOMAS ZGONIS, DPM, FACFAS
Director, Podiatric Surgical Residency and Reconstructive Fellowship Program; Chief, Division of Podiatric Medicine and Surgery, Associate Professor, Department of Orthopedic Surgery, The University of Texas Health Science Center at San Antonio, San Antonio, Texas

Contents

Pediatric Heel Pain   **355**

Warren A. Chiodo and Keith D. Cook

> Heel pain is a condition that is generally more common in the adult population. However, it is a condition that the foot and ankle specialist must be prepared to treat in pediatric patients. The insidious onset of heel pain in the pediatric patient can be an enigma to the foot and ankle specialist. Some of the more common etiologies for pediatric heel pain are discussed. The presenting signs and symptoms, as well as proper workup and treatment are discussed. Two case reports of unusual pediatric calcaneal fractures are also presented.

Plantar Fasciitis: Current Diagnostic Modalities and Treatments   **369**

Kevin Healey and Katherine Chen

> Plantar fasciitis is a common cause of heel pain. The diagnosis is made clinically and validated with different diagnostic modalities ranging from ultrasound to magnetic resonance imaging. Treatments vary from stretching exercises to different surgical options. No single treatment is guaranteed to alleviate the heel pain.

Internal and External Fixation Approaches to the Surgical Management of Calcaneal Fractures   **381**

John J. Stapleton, Gennady Kolodenker, and Thomas Zgonis

> Calcaneal fractures are one of the most difficult fractures to surgically manage and often require a steep learning curve to achieve consistent results. They usually occur in young individuals with labor intensive occupations and are associated with major complications. Conservative treatment of intraarticular calcaneal fractures with displacement often results in significant deformity, bone loss, and posttraumatic arthrosis. Optimally, an open approach is required in most cases to achieve anatomic reduction and successful long-term outcomes.

Complications of Heel Surgery   **393**

George F. Wallace

> Surgical complications of the calcaneus are unique to that structure but do not have a greater incidence than in any other part of the foot or ankle. The first tenet of any complication, however, is to recognize it. When all is said and done, recognition is probably the most important step when a complication arises.

a challenge for reconstructive surgeons. Posttraumatic composite bone and soft tissue defects are usually the result of high-energy trauma and are often associated with concomitant injuries, therefore making complex reconstruction more difficult. This article presents a case report of an open distal tibial fracture managed by a simultaneous distraction osteogenesis and Papineau technique with a long term follow-up and literature review.

Acute compartment syndrome is a known possible complication of calcaneal fractures and few case reports have documented a recurrent event after initial surgical fasciotomies. This article describes a rare case demonstrating a recurrence of acute compartment syndrome within days of initial fasciotomies and surgical repair of a comminuted calcaneal fracture.

RELATED INTEREST

Foot and Ankle Clinics Volume 15, Issue 1 (March 2010)
Traumatic Foot and Ankle Injuries Related to Recent International Conflicts
Edited by Eric Bluman, MD and James Ficke, MD

THE CLINICS ARE NOW AVAILABLE ONLINE!

Access your subscription at:
www.theclinics.com

Foreword

Heel Pain

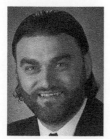

Thomas Zgonis, DPM, FACFAS
Consulting Editor

One of the most common problems encountered in our daily practices is heel pain. From pediatric to adult pathology, a wide range of conditions affecting the heel is seen, including neurogenic, biomechanical, inflammatory, neoplastic, or traumatic conditions. Malposition or malformation of the calcaneus typically results in devastating foot and ankle compensatory deformities while significantly altering the gait cycle. In addition, fractures of the calcaneus often pose great challenges to treating surgeons and, unfortunately, all too often anatomic reductions do not always lead to successful functional outcomes. A significant amount still needs to be learned in regards to how various conditions, deformities, and fracture patterns of the calcaneus are treated and managed.

This issue brings together a wide panel of experts in treating any type of heel pathology. I would like to commend the selected authors for providing readers with informative, innovative, and novel approaches to some of the most challenging case scenarios. I would also like to thank our guest editor, Dr George Wallace, for putting this issue together and for sharing his knowledge and tremendous experience as a leader in the field of foot and ankle academia, truly evident throughout this issue.

Thomas Zgonis, DPM, FACFAS
Division of Podiatric Medicine and Surgery
Department of Orthopaedic Surgery
The University of Texas Health Science Center at San Antonio
7703 Floyd Curl Drive–MSC 7776, San Antonio
TX 78229, USA

E-mail address:
zgonis@uthscsa.edu

Clin Podiatr Med Surg 27 (2010) xiii
doi:10.1016/j.cpm.2010.05.002   **podiatric.theclinics.com**
0891-8422/10/$ – see front matter © 2010 Elsevier Inc. All rights reserved.

Preface

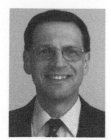

George F. Wallace, DPM, MBA
Guest Editor

Welcome to this issue of *Clinics in Podiatric Medicine and Surgery*. The authors have compiled articles dealing with heel pain from unique perspectives. However, no issue on heel pain would be complete without dealing with plantar fasciitis; therefore, this topic serves as the foundational article. Most heel pain ultimately is diagnosed as plantar fasciitis. As physicians, we never want to think all heel pain is fascial in origin. Systemic causes can masquerade as plantar fasciitis. Hoof beats may not always be horses. The words "index of suspicion" are three words that aid in our ability to differentiate who or what is causing the hoof beats.[1] I would like to thank all of the authors who are associated with University Hospital – University of Medicine and Dentistry of New Jersey and painstakingly worked to see this issue arrive at your desk. May you enjoy reading this issue of *Clinics in Podiatric Medicine and Surgery* and come away with learning at least one fact from each article that may improve your care of the patient with heel pain.

George F. Wallace, DPM, MBA
Podiatry Service
University Hospital – University of Medicine and Dentistry of New Jersey
150 Bergen Street, G-142, Newark, NJ 07103, USA

E-mail address:
wallacgf@umdnj.edu

REFERENCE

1. Groopman J. How doctors think. Boston: Houghton Mifflin Company; 2007.

Clin Podiatr Med Surg 27 (2010) xv
doi:10.1016/j.cpm.2010.05.001
0891-8422/10/$ – see front matter © 2010 Elsevier Inc. All rights reserved.

podiatric.theclinics.com

Pediatric Heel Pain

Warren A. Chiodo, DPM, Keith D. Cook, DPM*

KEYWORDS

- Pediatric • Heel • Calcaneus • Pain
- Calcaneal apophysitis • Fracture

Foot pain is an uncommon finding within the pediatric population. Heel pain, in particular, is far less common in children than it is in the adult population. Although pain is not commonly reported as a chief complaint, parents will often state that their children limp, walk on their toes, want to be carried instead of walking, are unable to keep up with their peers, or complain of fatigue in the feet.

Pediatric heel pain may begin following an acute traumatic event or have an insidious onset. Whether running through the house, learning to ride a bicycle, or participating in sporting activities, children can develop heel pain at some time in their young lives. Gathering a comprehensive history from a pediatric patient can be a daunting task. The child's parents or guardian are essential in obtaining an accurate history of the events that have led to the pediatric heel pain. Knowledge of the differential diagnoses affecting the pediatric heel can assist the podiatric physician in formulating a treatment plan to bring about a successful resolution of the problem so that children can return to their level of activity without detriment to their continued growth.

Pediatric heel pain can be a complex problem with many factors. These factors can include but are not limited to history of recent trauma, shoe gear, biomechanics, childhood development, or physical activities on various playing surfaces. This article provides an overview of several differential diagnoses for the painful pediatric heel. The framework of diagnosing and treating various etiologies of pediatric heel pain are provided for the foot and ankle specialist.

PEDIATRIC HEEL ANATOMY

At the time of birth, the calcaneus is mostly cartilaginous with ossification beginning at the primary growth center within the calcaneal tuberosity. A secondary growth center at the apophysis located posterior to the tuberosity is also present. As ossification continues and the calcaneus develops, cartilage remains between the body of the calcaneus and the apophysis. This separation exists until the end of puberty, generally

This work was not supported by any grants or outside funding.
Podiatry Service, University Hospital-University of Medicine and Dentistry of New Jersey, 150 Bergen Street, Room G-142, Newark, NJ 07103, USA
* Corresponding author.
E-mail address: cookkd@umdnj.edu

about the age of 14 in females and16 in males. The apophysis is also the site of attachment for fibers from the Achilles tendon as well as the plantar fascia.

CALCANEAL APOPHYSITIS

In 1912, J.W. Sever first reported calcaneal apophysitis as an inflammation of the apophysis causing pain to the heel, mild swelling, and difficulty walking.[1] Calcaneal apophysitis is commonly thought of as the most common osteochondrosis occurring in the pediatric foot.[2] It is associated with heel pain in children, generally between the ages of 8 and 14, who are physically active. Historically, calcaneal apophysitis was much more common in young males compared with females, although this trend may not be as relevant today with more young females being involved in sports.

Calcaneal apophysitis is characterized by dull, achy pain located in the posterior and plantar aspects of the heel. Pain is generally present after periods of prolonged activity or upon beginning activity after rest (poststatic dyskinesia). An antalgic gait including limping, tiptoeing, or walking on the outside of the foot may be a chief complaint on presentation. On physical examination, pain can be elicited with direct palpation of the apophysis or with medial to lateral compression of the heel. Pain can also be elicited with dorsiflexion of the ankle. A common finding associated with pediatric calcaneal apophysitis is gastrocnemius-soleus complex equinus.[3]

Radiographically, calcaneal apophysitis cannot definitively be diagnosed or ruled out because of normal anatomic variations. Often, plain-film radiographs of a pediatric patient with calcaneal apophysitis will demonstrate sclerotic changes, fragmentation, or a combination of sclerosis and fragmentation of the apophysis (**Fig. 1**).

In a study by Volpon and de Carvalho Filho,[4] the calcanei of 392 children with no complaints of heel pain and 69 children with a diagnosis of calcaneal apophysitis were evaluated radiographically. They reported that the sclerotic aspect of the apophysis was a normal variation, which should not be used to confirm or deny a diagnosis of calcaneal apophysitis. However, they found that the degree of fragmentation of the apophysis was greater in the group that had a diagnosis of calcaneal apophysitis. They extrapolated that the degree of fragmentation may be suggestive of a mechanical etiology for the condition.

With the advent of magnetic resonance imaging (MRI), several theories to explain the insidious onset of pediatric heel pain have been developed. One theory looks to explain pediatric heel pain not as an overuse injury of the apophysis, but rather as a stress fracture of the calcaneal metaphysis immediately adjacent to the region of the apophysis.

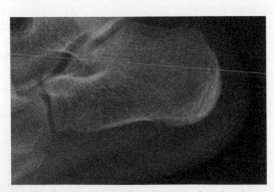

Fig. 1. Lateral radiograph of a 12-year-old boy diagnosed with calcaneal apophysitis.

Ogden and colleagues[5] performed MRI studies on children with a presumptive diagnosis of calcaneal apophysitis. The MRI studies demonstrated evidence of bone bruising within the metaphyseal region of the calcaneus in close proximity to the calcaneal apophysis with minimal signal changes seen in the apophysis itself. Follow-up MRI studies performed after treatment with immobilization showed decreased signal intensity within the metaphyseal bone with minimal change to the signal intensity in the apophysis. Accordingly, the MRI findings were coupled with improvement of clinical symptoms. The possibility of increased signal changes being nothing more than bone bruising could not be excluded.

The authors of this article believe that calcaneal apophysitis is an overuse injury resulting in abnormal biologic stresses applied to the calcaneus as a whole without distinction of apophyseal versus metaphyseal injury. The nomenclature and description of calcaneal apophysitis as an inflammatory disorder of the calcaneal apophysis is an outdated and disproven theory based on failure of anti-inflammatory medications alone to relieve symptomatology, as well as advances in the imaging of the calcaneus in pediatric patients diagnosed with the condition of a painful heel.[5]

Treatment of calcaneal apophysitis has long been a source of debate. The need for complete immobilization with casting is not always necessary for treatment of this condition. Often, the choice of protected, partial weight bearing for 2 to 4 weeks as necessary depending on the severity of the symptoms is preferred. The authors' preferred course of therapy consists of placing the patient in a CAM-walker and instituting partial weight bearing for approximately 2 weeks with the assistance of crutches. During this 2-week period, the lower extremity is rested to allow any symptoms to subside. The offending activity is eliminated during the recovery period. Analgesics or anti-inflammatory medication may also be used as deemed necessary by the clinician. If symptomatic relief is achieved after 2 weeks, patients are advised to begin a stretching protocol, which will be described in the latter portion of this section. At this time, patients may be progressed to weight bearing as tolerated in regular shoe gear with limitation of physical activities. If symptoms persist, continued use of the CAM-walker is advised until symptoms have resolved.

A mainstay of treatment continues to be the stretching and elongation of the gastrocnemius-soleal complex and by extension, the plantar fascia. Once the acute symptoms of the child's heel pain have resolved, a stretching protocol is initiated. The child is instructed to perform lower extremity stretching exercises 3 to 5 times per day. The protocol consists of passive dorsiflexion of the affected foot at the ankle with the use of a belt, towel, or Thera-Band (The Hygenic Corp, Akron, OH, USA)

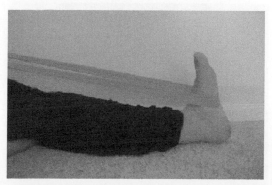

Fig. 2. Demonstration of seated gastrocnemius-soleal complex stretching with a towel.

(**Fig. 2**). This exercise is performed in a seated position with the knee extended. The patients are also instructed to perform Achilles tendon and calf stretches while standing and leaning into a wall with the affected heel firmly on the ground. This is performed with the knee extended on the affected limb and the contralateral limb in the flexed position (**Fig. 3**). Each stretching exercise should be performed using slow, controlled motions and held for approximately 10 seconds each time. Patients and their families are advised that increased amount and frequency of stretching generally correlate with better treatment outcomes and decreased incidence of recurrence. Should the patient's symptoms not improve, formal physical therapy may need to be instituted.

Upon complete relief of symptoms, patients are gradually reintroduced to their sporting activities. A modification of shoe gear such as changing from screw-in cleats to molded cleats may be required to allow for a change in cleat position. Orthotic devices may also be used to alter the biomechanics and shock absorption of the pediatric heel.

FOREIGN BODY

Another source of pediatric heel pain is a retained foreign body. Pediatric patients and their parents will generally present to an office or emergency room complaining of a painful heel after stepping on "something." However, in very young patients, a limp on the affected side may be the presenting complaint. Upon examination, tenderness to palpation at the site of entry may be present. Depending on the duration of time between injury and presentation, the entry wound may be difficult to find. An area of erythema may be present depending on the immune response of the surrounding body tissue and the reactivity of the foreign body present.

In the authors' experience, the foreign bodies likely to be encountered include, but are not limited to, glass, splinters, pins, or sewing needles. Glass is often encountered when a patient reports experiencing pain after running around outdoors without shoe gear. Sewing needles are often found in patients who are barefoot within the home, usually on a carpeted surface (**Fig. 4**). Splinters, unlike glass and needles, can be encountered either indoors or outdoors because of hardwood flooring and hardwood decks.

Following a thorough history and physical, radiographs should be obtained to ensure no bony involvement, particularly if infection is present or significant time has elapsed since entry of the foreign body. Depending on the location of the object

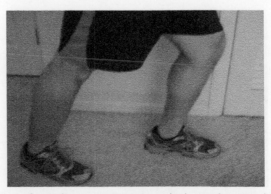

Fig. 3. Demonstration of standing gastrocnemius-soleal complex stretching.

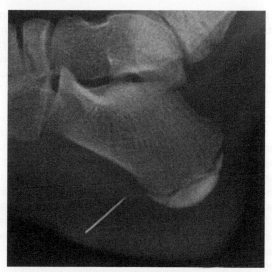

Fig. 4. Lateral radiograph showing a metallic foreign body plantar to the calcaneus in an 8-year-old girl.

within the rear foot and the material of the object, anteroposterior and oblique views may be of little value in locating the object. On the other hand, the lateral and calcaneal axial views are often useful in determining location as well as orientation of the object, which may be of significant benefit when it comes to removing the foreign body.

In instances where the object is wood or glass, radiographs may not be helpful. In certain settings, further evaluation of glass or wooden objects with ultrasound may prove more effective than plain radiographs. However, it is important to note that ultrasound is user dependent and may be an exercise in futility because of the orientation of the transducer to the object. False negatives may be encountered if the transducer and object are oriented within the same plane and no object is observed.

Treatment for foreign bodies retained in the heel includes proper tetanus prophylaxis, removal of the foreign body with irrigation of the wound, and possible antibiotic therapy. The authors' protocol for removal of foreign bodies includes use of local anesthetic to the affected area followed by prepping and draping of the affected foot using standard aseptic technique. Mini C-Arm radiography may be used to locate the position and orientation of the foreign body if the material of the foreign body lends itself to radiographic examination.

Removal of the foreign body is then attempted for a minimum of 30 minutes. If the foreign body cannot be removed after 30 minutes, formal incision and drainage in an operating room may be necessary.

After successful removal of the foreign body, irrigation with a combination of povidone-iodine solution and normal saline is then performed. To perform high-pressure irrigation of the wound, approximately 20 mL of irrigant is drawn into a 20-mL syringe that has an 18-gauge angio-catheter attached at the tip. A minimum of 60 mL of irrigant is required for proper irrigation of the wound. The entry site wound is then packed open to allow for drainage. A dry sterile dressing and compressive wrap are applied. Weight bearing as tolerated in a postoperative shoe is allowed. However, in many cases, pain may prohibit weight bearing and the use of crutches may be necessary.

Antibiotic therapy for foreign bodies encountered within the pediatric heel is a subject of debate with differing views offered in the literature. Often, the use of oral or parenteral antibiotics is dependent on the individual foot and ankle specialist based on the clinical signs and symptoms encountered as well as timing of the injury. In a report by Weber,[6] the incidence of infection following plantar puncture wounds was found to be 6.4%, regardless of whether or not the wounds were evaluated by a physician. When excluding wounds that were not seen by a physician, the calculated incidence of infection rose to 11.4%, possibly indicating that only the more severe wounds are seen by physicians.

If the foreign body is removed and no signs of infection (ie, erythema, cellulitis, purulence, calor, edema) are present, oral antibiotic therapy is generally not indicated. If a retained foreign body is present for longer than 8 hours or signs of infection are present, oral antibiotic therapy is indicated. Antibiotic therapy focuses on common bacterial pathogens known to cause skin and soft tissue infections, mainly *Staphylococcus* species and *Streptococcus* species. At the authors' institution, cephalexin administered in the appropriate dosage dependent on the pediatric patient for 7 days is used for patients with no known allergy to penicillin or cephalosporins. In patients with a known penicillin or cephalosporin allergy, trimethoprim-sulfamethoxazole (Bactrim) or clindamycin, in the proper pediatric dosages, are used.

Following treatment in the acute setting, patients are routinely followed in the University Hospital-UMDNJ Podiatry Center. It is important to remember that, although the initial problem was treated successfully, sequelae to the foreign body can occur including but not limited to inclusion cysts and verrucae. These conditions are commonly encountered subsequent to a foreign body because of the puncture wound. A severe complication following foreign body injuries is direct extension osteomyelitis, which should be prevented at all times. These conditions may also lead to pediatric heel pain as well.

TUMORS

In many instances, heel pain in the pediatric population is a result of biomechanical forces. In rare instances, however, pediatric heel pain can result from the development of calcaneal bone tumors. Malignant tumors that can cause pediatric heel pain include osteosarcoma, Ewing's sarcoma, and chondrosarcoma. Some benign tumors known to affect the pediatric heel include unicameral bone cysts, aneurysmal bone cysts (ABCs), giant cell tumors, osteoid osteomas, osteoblastomas, and nonossifying fibromas. However, it is beyond the scope of this article to explore each of these tumors in detail.

Whether benign or malignant, evaluation for bone tumors is performed by first obtaining standard radiographs with particular emphasis on location of the pain. Many lesions are commonly seen in the metaphyseal region of the bone. Evaluation for cortical disruption and periosteal reactions can often be key indicators as to the aggressiveness of the lesion and whether the tumor is malignant or benign. MRI studies are also obtained to evaluate the lesions and their possible extension into the soft tissues surrounding the calcaneus.

In cases of benign tumors, symptomatic relief may be achieved by the use of anti-inflammatory medicines. This is particularly true for the osteoid osteoma, where a key characteristic is pain relief with salicylates. Surgical intervention is generally warranted only when the lesions are symptomatic or may lead to pathologic fracture.[7] In cases where surgical intervention is indicated, curettage and filling of the resultant defects with bone graft material has been found to be effective. In a study by Dormans and colleagues,[8] all 24 patients included in the study were able to return to full activity and were asymptomatic following surgical management for unicameral bone cysts. Serial radiographs are generally obtained to evaluate for any regrowth of the tumor.

If a malignant tumor is encountered in the pediatric patient, it is advised that consultation with a pediatric orthopedic oncologist be obtained before any intervention. Once a full workup for spread of the malignancy is performed and found to be negative, treatment of solitary lower extremity lesions can be performed including excision of the tumor with appropriate resection of surrounding margins. If malignancy is found to exist, all future intervention should be referred to the pediatric oncologist for appropriate treatment that may include surgical resection, amputation, chemotherapy, radiation therapy, or any combination of these therapies.

FRACTURES

Pediatric calcaneal fractures are fairly uncommon with a low reported incidence when compared with adult calcaneal fractures. However, the calcaneus is the most commonly fractured tarsal bone in pediatric patients. The incidence of pediatric calcaneal fractures may be low because of missed diagnoses, low referral rates to appropriate physicians, or low index of suspicion for a calcaneal fracture. This low index of suspicion can lead to a delay in seeking medical attention at which time the healing process has already begun and the injury may be almost healed.[9]

Pediatric heel fractures can be subdivided into traumatic fractures and stress fractures. Traumatic pediatric calcaneal fractures result from similar mechanisms of injury as adult calcaneal fractures, including motor vehicle accidents, a fall from a height, or other blunt force injury. Wiley and Profitt[10] reported that in pediatric patients younger than 10, a simple fall possessed enough force to cause a fracture. Although increased fall heights often lead to more significant adult calcaneal fractures with comminution, such correlations have not been noted in the pediatric population.[11]

Stress fractures of the pediatric heel occur secondary to repetitive microtrauma. This microtrauma can be as a result of repetitive motions, particularly in children engaged in athletic activities. Commonly, stress fractures are encountered in sports played on harder surfaces like basketball, volleyball, or tennis. It is important to remember that shoe gear can also play a role in stress fracture formation. Certain athletic shoes, particularly shoes with cleats, may lead to stress fracture formation of the heel because of the location of the cleat under the heel (**Fig. 5**). The force caused by the repetitive trauma, if not properly distributed, is simply more stress than the pediatric calcaneus can sustain. Often, stress fractures are encountered in the tuberosity of the calcaneus.

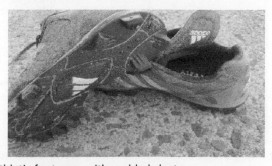

Fig. 5. Image of athletic foot gear with molded cleats.

As with any fracture, the choice of radiographic evaluation is a key part in diagnosis and treatment planning. At the authors' institution, radiographic protocol for all traumatic calcaneal fractures, pediatric and adult, includes standard foot views (anteroposterior, medial oblique, and lateral) and calcaneal axial views. Calcaneal axial views are beneficial in assessing the degree of varus angulation of the calcaneal tuberosity when a joint depression fracture is present. If a fracture Is suspected or evident on plain film, computed tomography (CT) scans in the coronal, axial, and sagittal planes are also obtained. MRI studies are reserved for cases of suspected stress fractures of the calcaneus.

Because of the morphology of the pediatric heel, specifically the ratio of cartilage to bone, initial plain radiographs do not often demonstrate a clear fracture line and may be read as negative.[12,13] Subsequent radiographs taken 10 to 14 days later may reveal evidence of a healing fracture, depicted by calcification or sclerosis along the fracture line. In addition, because of the largely cartilaginous nature of the calcaneus, it is difficult to locate the bony landmarks necessary to accurately assess Bohler's angle and the critical angle of Gissane in children younger than 10.[14,15]

Because of the difficulties viewing calcaneal fractures on standard radiographs, advanced imaging should always be obtained. Use of CT scans should be standard in evaluating calcaneal fractures of traumatic origin in the pediatric population. As with adult calcaneal fractures, CT scans are superior in demonstrating involvement of the posterior facet, sustentaculum tali, or calcaneo-cubiod joint and the amount of comminution. Rotation of fracture fragments is also clearly visualized with the use of CT scans. The Sanders classification is widely accepted for pediatric calcaneal fractures because of its prognostic value.

Although CT scans are preferred for traumatic fractures of the pediatric heel, MRI studies are preferred when a stress fracture of the pediatric heel is suspected. Whereas standard radiographs will demonstrate evidence of fracture healing after approximately 10 to 14 days, MRI can lead to the quicker diagnosis of a stress fracture and initiation of treatment. On T2-weighted imaging, a stress fracture will present as an area of increased signal intensity representing bone marrow edema (**Fig. 6**).

Nonoperative management for traumatic pediatric calcaneal fractures is indicated when there is less than 2 mm of disruption of the 3 subtalar joints (posterior, middle,

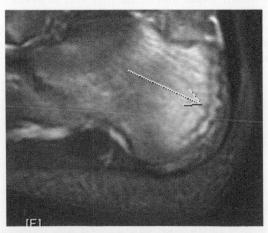

Fig. 6. MRI image showing a stress fracture of the calcaneus with surrounding bone marrow edema.

and anterior facets), no subtalar joint subluxation/dislocation, and no fibular impingement from the lateral cortex of the calcaneus. Tongue-type fractures can also be managed nonoperatively when the posterior gap is less than 2 mm and there is no significant shortening of the Achilles tendon secondary to proximal migration of the fracture fragment. In addition, extensive soft tissue damage needs to be appropriately managed before proceeding with surgical intervention.

The Podiatry Department at University Hospital-UMDNJ initiates conservative treatment of acute traumatic and stress fractures of the calcaneus by placing the affected lower extremity in a Jones compressive dressing consisting of cast padding and compressive wraps. A posterior splint is then applied to the extremity with the ankle in neutral position. In cases of uncontrollable pain or pain out of proportion with the injury, a compartment syndrome needs to be evaluated and treated accordingly. In the more usual case where no compartment syndrome is present, the patient is instructed to remain non–weight bearing to the affected limb with use of crutches, with elevation of the extremity, and ice to the affected limb. The patient is then evaluated weekly. Once the edema has subsided, the patient is placed into a well-padded below-knee fiberglass cast for 4 to 6 weeks. During this time the patient continues to be non–weight bearing. Repeat radiographic examination is performed after that time and the patient may be progressed to partial weight bearing in a CAM-walker when fracture healing is noted radiographically. The patient is transitioned to full weight bearing and normal shoe gear as tolerated.

Open reduction with internal fixation of traumatic pediatric calcaneal fractures is a reasonable option when the amount of displacement exceeds that listed previously or there is joint incongruity. The goals of treatment for pediatric patients are the same as those for adults. They include restoration of the articular surfaces of the subtalar and calcaneo-cuboid joints, restoration of calcaneal height and width, and restoration of the lateral wall of the calcaneus. In one study by Pickle and colleagues,[16] open reduction with internal fixation was performed for displaced intra-articular calcaneal fractures in 6 pediatric patients with good short-term results and no development of serious complications encountered when compared with adult patients undergoing similar procedures.

CASE REPORTS
Case 1: Calcaneal Stress Fracture

A 14-year-old male presented with his father to the University Hospital-UMDNJ Podiatry Center complaining of right lower extremity pain in the area of the Achilles tendon for approximately 2 weeks. The patient stated that it occurred after running during lacrosse practice in a pair of hi-top sneakers rather than his usual running shoes. The patient denied feeling or hearing a "pop" suggestive of an Achilles tendon rupture. After the onset of pain, both the patient and the patient's father stated he had altered his gait, placing weight on the outside of the foot. Conservative therapy was initiated by the high school athletic trainer consisting of stretching and ice baths after practices.

Following a thorough history, the physical examination was performed. The vascular examination revealed palpable pedal pulses bilaterally, normal capillary refill time to all digits, and no significant edema. Neurologic examination revealed epicritic sensation to be intact. Attention was then focused to the area of concern just proximal to the insertion of the Achilles tendon where pain on palpation was noted with no palpable dell suggestive of tendon rupture. No pain could be elicited on palpation or compression of the patient's calcaneus. Full muscle strength was noted with active plantarflexion on the affected limb, which was comparable to the contralateral limb. Gait analysis revealed compensatory ambulation on the lateral aspect of the right foot with an early heel lift.

At this time, the presumptive diagnoses included a partial tear of the Achilles tendon, Achilles tendonitis, or tendonosis. The patient was placed into a CAM-walker and allowed to bear weight as tolerated. The patient and his father were instructed to obtain an MRI of the right ankle and rearfoot before the next clinic visit.

MRI of the right ankle and rearfoot revealed no abnormality within the Achilles tendon, its sheath, or in any of the soft tissues surrounding the ankle joint/rearfoot complex. However, a linear focus of signal intensity was seen on T2-weighted imaging. This focus of signal intensity was noted within the metaphysis of the calcaneus adjacent to the apophysis surrounded by bone marrow edema (**Fig. 7**). A diagnosis of calcaneal stress fracture was made based on the physical examination and MRI results.

At follow-up, the examination revealed a decrease in pain at the Achilles tendon of the right lower extremity. Unlike the previous visit, pain was now elicited with side-to-side compression of the calcaneus distal to the apophysis. The patient was placed in a short-leg cast and instructed to remain non–weight bearing with use of crutches for 4 weeks and obtain new radiographs before the next visit. After 1 month of casting and non–weight bearing, the patient returned to the University Hospital-UMDNJ Podiatry Center and had the cast removed. Repeat physical examination at this time revealed no pain to the right foot or ankle. Standard radiographs showed no evidence of fracture. The patient was progressed to partial weight bearing on the right lower extremity in the CAM-walker for 1 week and instructed to bear weight as tolerated in the CAM-walker after the first week. The patient returned 3 weeks later, having spent the preceding 2 weeks full weight bearing on the right foot. Repeat radiographs remained negative. Two weeks later, the patient remained pain free while ambulating in regular shoe gear and was allowed to return to lacrosse and his normal activities.

Case 2: Intra-articular Calcaneal Fracture

An 8-year-old male presented to University Hospital-UMDNJ 4 days status post an injury to his right foot in which he slipped and tripped over a soccer ball. The patient stated that he was unable to walk on the right foot immediately after sustaining the injury.

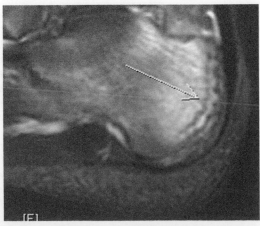

Fig. 7. MRI image showing a stress fracture of the calcaneus in a 15-year-old boy.

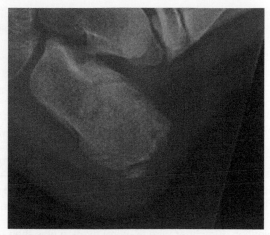

Fig. 8. Lateral radiograph showing a calcaneal fracture in a 9-year-old boy.

After a thorough history was illicited, a complete physical examination was performed for the lower extremities bilaterally. The patient was found to have palpable pedal pulses, intact sensation to the toes, and intact motor function with ability to move the digits. Standard radiographs demonstrated a right calcaneal fracture **(Fig. 8)**. Per the authors' protocol, CT scans were obtained of the involved foot and a 3-part intra-articular calcaneal fracture with joint depression of the posterior facet was noted **(Fig. 9)**. The patient was placed in a Jones compressive dressing with a well-padded posterior splint to the right lower extremity.

After being appropriately optimized, the patient underwent open reduction with internal fixation of the fracture. The fracture was approached through an S-shaped skin incision overlying the lateral aspect of the sinus tarsi, which was carried down to the level of bone. The height of the posterior facet was restored and visualized under

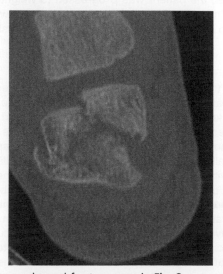

Fig. 9. CT scan of the same calcaneal fracture seen in **Fig. 8**.

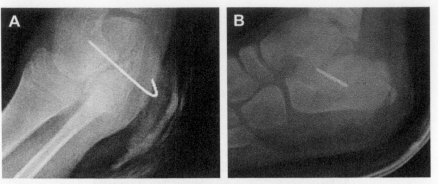

Fig. 10. (*A, B*) Postoperative radiographs depicting K-wire fixation of the calcaneal fracture previously seen in **Figs. 8** and **9**.

fluoroscopic examination. Kirschner wire (K-wire) fixation was then used to fixate the posterior facet fragment to the sustentaculum tali (**Fig. 10**). A defect was noted in the region of the neutral triangle and was filled with demineralized bone matrix. A temporary Steinman pin was placed through the medial aspect of the calcaneus and used to correct the varus rotation to the calcaneal tuberosity. Standard tissue closure was performed and a dry sterile dressing and well-padded posterior splint were applied to the right lower extremity.

Following the procedure, the patient was instructed to remain non–weight bearing to the right lower extremity using crutches. The patient followed up in the University Hospital-UMDNJ Podiatry Center approximately 1 week after surgery. At this time, a well-padded below-knee cast was applied and non–weight bearing to the right lower extremity using crutches was continued because of adequate wound healing and edema control. Radiographs taken 4 weeks postoperative showed interval healing with K-wire fixation remaining intact. At this time, the cast was removed, the K-wire extracted, and the patient was progressed to non–weight bearing in a CAM-walker using crutches. Range of motion exercises were initiated at this time as well. Upon follow-up 2 weeks later, the patient was progressed to weight bearing as tolerated in regular shoe gear. The patient's postoperative course was without complications. The patient returned to his preinjury activity level 5 months postoperatively.

SUMMARY

Many factors can lead to the development of heel pain in the pediatric patient. It is up to the podiatric physician to investigate and correctly identify the agent responsible for causing the condition known as pediatric heel pain. Discussed are several common causes of pediatric heel pain including calcaneal apophysitis, calcaneal fractures, foreign bodies, and bone tumors. Each condition requires appropriate evaluation and management to alleviate the symptoms and return pediatric patients to their optimum level of activity while preventing any detriment to their continued growth. Whether conservative or surgical, treatment protocols have been established with this goal in mind. In formulating treatment plans, it is important that podiatric physicians couple the understanding of the etiologies of the condition with the most sophisticated technologies available to make their diagnoses. The current environment of evidence-based medicine should continue to lead the way to formulating proper, effective protocols that disregard unproven treatment options that can be costly, both in money and in time.

REFERENCES

1. Sever JW. Apophysitis of the os calcis. N Y State J Med 1912;95:1025–9.
2. Macnicol M, Thomson P. Orthopedic conditions affecting the foot in childhood. Introduction to Podopediatrics. New York: Elsevier; 2001. p. 212–3.
3. Micheli LJ, Ireland ML. Prevention and management of calcaneal apophysitis in children: an overuse syndrome. J Pediatr Orthop 1987;7:34–8.
4. Volpon JB, de Carvalho Filho G. Calcaneal apophysitis: a quantitative radiographic evaluation of the secondary ossification center. Arch Orthop Trauma Surg 2002;122:338–41.
5. Ogden JA, Ganey T, Hill JD, et al. Sever's injury: a stress fracture of the immature calcaneal metaphysic. J Pediatr Orthop 2004;24(5):488–92.
6. Weber EJ. Plantar puncture wounds: a survey to determine the incidence of infection. J Accid Emerg Med 1996;13(4):274–7.
7. Ishikawa SN. Conditions of the calcaneus in skeletally immature patients. Foot Ankle Clin 2005;10(3):503–13.
8. Dormans JP, Sankar WN, Moroz L, et al. Percutaneous intramedullary decompression, curettage, and grafting with medical grade calcium sulfate pellets for unicameral bone cysts in children: a new minimally invasive technique. J Pediatr Orthop 2005;25(6):804–11.
9. Jarvis JG, Moroz PJ. Fractures and dislocations of the foot. In: Beatty JH , Kasser JR, editors. Rockwood and Wilkins' Fractures in children, 6th edition. New York: Lippincott Williams and Wilkins; 2006. p. 1144–55.
10. Wiley JJ, Profitt A. Fractures of the os calcis in children. Clin Orthop 1984;188: 131.
11. Atkins RM, Allen PE, Livingstone JA. Demographic features of intra-articular fractures of the calcaneum. Foot Ankle Surg 2001;7:77–84.
12. Inokuchi S, Usami N, Hiraishi E, et al. Calcaneal fractures in children. J Pediatr Orthop 1998;18(4):469–74.
13. Schantz K, Rasmussen F. Good prognosis after calcaneal fracture in children. Acta Orthop Scand 1988;59:560–3.
14. Howard CB, Benson MK. The ossific nuclei and the cartilage anlage of the talus and calcaneum. J Bone Joint Surg Br 1992;74:620–3.
15. Hubbard AM, Meyer JS, Davidson RS, et al. Relationship between the ossification center and cartilaginous anlage in the normal hindfoot in children: study with MR imaging. Am J Roentgenol 1993;161:849–53.
16. Pickle A, Benaroch T, Guy P, et al. Clinical outcome of pediatric calcaneal fractures treated with open reduction and internal fixation. J Pediatr Orthop 2004; 24(2):178–80.

Plantar Fasciitis: Current Diagnostic Modalities and Treatments

Kevin Healey, DPM*, Katherine Chen, DPM

KEYWORDS

• Plantar fasciitis • Foot • Heel pain

Plantar fasciitis is one of the most common causes of heel pain seen by foot and ankle surgeons. Approximately 10% to 16% of the population suffer from plantar fasciitis.[1] This is usually an overuse injury at the origin of the plantar fascia caused by excessive stress to the foot or biomechanical abnormalities of the foot such as excessive pronation. This condition may cause inflammatory or degenerative changes of the fascia and periostitis of the medial calcaneal tubercle.

Bilateral plantar fasciitis may be caused by arthridides such as rheumatoid arthritis, Reiter disease, ankylosing spondylitis, systemic lupus erythematosus, and gout.

ANATOMY

The plantar fascia, or plantar aponeurosis, is predominantly composed of longitudinal collagen fibers that start at the anterior aspect of the calcaneal tubercle, extend distally into 5 digital bands at the metatarsophalangeal joints, and terminate at the dorsal aspect of the proximal phalanges. The fibers blend into the dermis, flexor tendon sheaths, deep transverse metatarsal ligaments, and other ligament structures. The plantar fascia consists of 3 bands: medial, central, and lateral. Each band is separated by an intermuscular septum that splits the intrinsic plantar muscle into their different compartments.

The lateral band is superficial to the abductor digiti quinti minimi muscle. It is also attached to the lateral process of the calcaneus and the base of the fifth metatarsal. The medial band of the plantar fascia is superficial to the abductor hallucis muscle. This band is connected to the flexor retinaculum. The flexor digitorum brevis muscle arises from the central band of the plantar fascia.

University Hospital, University of Medicine and Dentistry of New Jersey, 150 Bergen Street, Newark, NJ, USA
* Corresponding author.
E-mail address: healeykm@hotmail.com

Clin Podiatr Med Surg 27 (2010) 369–380
doi:10.1016/j.cpm.2010.03.002
0891-8422/10/$ – see front matter © 2010 Elsevier Inc. All rights reserved.

podiatric.theclinics.com

The plantar fascial bands are supplied by the medial and lateral plantar nerves. The thickness of a normal plantar fascia is approximately 3 mm. In patients with plantar fasciitis, the maximum thickness is significantly increased to 7 mm.[2]

DEFINITION

Plantar fasciitis is described as a painful inflammatory process, generally at the origin of the plantar fascia on the calcaneus. It can also be central in the plantar arch, or, less commonly, distal.[3] Lemont and colleagues[4] state that the disorder is better classified as a fasciosis rather than a fasciitis, with chronic degeneration of the plantar fascia rather than a true itis or inflammatory condition.

RISK FACTORS

Plantar fasciitis is often seen in patients between the ages of 40 and 60 years. It is more common in women. Occupations that require people to walk a lot or stand on hard surfaces for long periods of time can also damage the plantar fascia. The condition is common in athletes, nurses, letter carriers, warehouse workers, and auto mechanics.[1] Poor footwear, such as those that are thin soled, loose, or lack an arch support, can also contribute to plantar fasciitis.

Patients who are overweight or obese carry a larger force per unit area on their feet. This causes increased strain on the fascia, leading to chronic stretching with degeneration, and thus pain. Plantar fasciitis is also seen in pregnancy, with the weight gain over a short period of time causing increased stress on the ligamentous structures of the foot.

Decrease in ankle dorsiflexion is another risk factor for plantar fasciitis.[1] Normal gait requires a minimum 10° of dorsiflexion at the ankle joint to clear the ground. If the patient has less than 10° of dorsiflexion, the foot will compensate by pronating and increasing the tensile load on the plantar fascia.

SYMPTOMS

Pain is usually localized to the medial calcaneal tubercle, but can be distal and along the entire length of the fascia. In the acute phase of plantar fasciitis, pain is sharp and worse with the first step of the day after a period of non–weight bearing. This is known as poststatic dyskinesia. Pain initially improves after a few steps or minutes, but then worsens with additional weight bearing. In the chronic stages, pain is dull and constant. The fascia has been inflamed, healed, and then stressed again with continuous weight bearing. This process leads to chronic degenerative changes to the fasica. Histologically, collagen necrosis, giofibroplastic hyperplasia, chondroid metaplasia, and matrix calcification are seen.[4]

PATHOMECHANICS

During stance, the medial longitudinal arch functions similarly to a truss, with tension along the plantar fascia, in connection with 2 compressive elements.[5] Stretching or spreading of the arch in weight bearing is prevented by tension of the plantar fascia, muscles, and ligaments, with compression of the bone structures of the arch. Thus the stiffness of the arch is in proportion to the stresses, or loads, applied. Hicks[6] proposed that low arches seen in pes planus resulted in increased tension within the fascia. Salathe[7] stated that the greatest tension occurred within the fascia at heel-off.

Hicks[6] compared the plantar fascia working with the digits with a windlass. As the toes dorsiflex, the plantar fascia tightens as it courses around the metatarsal heads, causing shortening of the fascia and increased tension. Activation of the windlass mechanism causes increase in stability of the arch and prepares the foot for the propulsive phase of gait.

In patients with shortening or tightening of the Achilles tendon (equinus), stress becomes greater in the plantar fascia as the heel elevates. Because many of these patients also present with digital contractures, loads are further increased within the plantar fascia as the toes are dorsiflexed. Carpenter and colleagues[8] stated that there can be a 6-mm change in length of the plantar fascia during gait, indicating the effect of ground forces on load within the fascia.

Plantar fasciitis can be associated with pes planus and pes cavus. In a study of 82 patients, Prichasuk[9] suggested that pes planus was an important factor in patients with plantar fasciitis. Fascial thickening in the pes cavus patient is correlated with sagittal arch mechanics and can influence the severity of symptoms. Because the fascia is tighter and thicker, shock is less dissipated in stance and gait, causing increased tension at the origin on the calcaneus.

DIFFERENTIAL DIAGNOSES

The following are included in any patient presenting with plantar calcaneal pain.

Rheumatoid Arthritis

Generally, rheumatoid arthritis attacks diarthrodial joints. Other sites of involvement include tendons, tendon sheaths, subchondral bone, bursae, and periarticular subcutaneous tissue. The rheumatoid patient may present with heel pain, also with poststatic dyskinesia.

The basis for this pain is an inflammatory reaction in the epiphyseal portion of the calcaneus. Epiphyseal bone is similar histologically to synovial tissue, with the inflammatory process causing osteitis and irregular osteolysis of cortical bone. Radiographs of the foot may show periostitis, osteolysis, and loss of radiopacity of the soft tissues surrounding the calcaneus.

In juvenile rheumatoid arthritis, the epiphyseal plate may be invaded by the ostetitis, causing cystic destruction of the epiphyseal plate. This can cause retardation of growth. Because local manifestations of rheumatoid arthritis in the foot respond well to nonsteroidal antiinflammatory drugs (NSAIDs) and corticosteroid injection, a good medical history is mandatory. This history should include other areas of joint pain, morning stiffness, and edema to periarticular tissues. In addition to radiographs, laboratory studies should be performed, including rheumatoid arthritis latex, and a complete blood count along with erythrocyte sedimentation rate.

Rheumatoid nodules are chronic inflammatory lesions that occur in the subcutaneous tissue, particularly in areas of mechanical pressure. Plantar and medial to the calcaneal tuberosity is a common area for presentation in the foot. There is palpable swelling and sensation of a mass in the early stages, and magnetic resonance imaging (MRI) may be required for diagnosis.

Reiter Syndrome

Reiter syndrome is a triad consisting of nongonococcal urethritis, arthritis, and conjunctivitis. Articular involvement usually involves weight-bearing joints, but can include the toes and plantar calcaneal tuberosity area. Presentation may vary. There may be mild inflammation, or significant signs including rubor, calor, and severe pain. Synovitis may be migratory but can be followed by a more severe and persistent inflammation. Diagnostic studies include radiographs of the foot and the lymphocyte antigen HLA-B27. Periostitis of the plantar surface of the calcaneus is estimated to occur in 20% of patients with Reiter syndrome.

Ankylosing Spondylitis

Ankylosing spondylitis is an inflammatory arthritis involving the axial skeleton and, in the later stages, diarthrodial joints. The primary tissue involved in the disease process is cartilage, especially fibrocartilage. Often there is osteitis of subchondral bone. Synovitis, with inflammation of the enthesis and periosteum, is a feature of the disease process. Five percent of patients with ankylosing spondylitis present with heel pain due to periositis and osteitis of the plantar calcaneus. Diagnostic studies should include lymphocyte antigen HLA-B27 and pedal radiographs.[10]

Osteomyelitis

The calcaneus is a frequent site for hematogenous osteomyelitis in the foot, especially in the pediatric patient. Presentation includes calor, edema, and pain with standing and walking. Fever and leukocytosis may accompany this presentation. Direct extension osteomyelitis is more common in the podiatric practice, especially in the diabetic patient. It is accompanied by an open lesion or ulceration and may include drainage, cellulitis, and systemic signs.

Radiographs of the foot show periostitis, erosion, and bony destruction. MRI may be performed in the early stages and may show osteomyelitis before any plain-film changes. Culture and sensitivity of purulence or drainage with subsequent bone culture are performed to confirm the diagnosis and plan treatment. Treatment plans may include intravenous antibiotics, irrigation and debridement, and subsequent planning for skin coverage.

Calcaneal Stress Fracture

Calcaneal stress fracture must be included in the differential diagnosis of heel pain. Patients present with diffuse swelling and ecchymosis, often after prolonged or significant activity. Lateral compression of the heel helps with the diagnosis. The calcaneus is prone to stress fracture because of its anatomy, with a thin cortical shell surrounding primarily cancellous bone. Patients involved in athletic activities or prolonged walking may feel a sharp pain with limited ability to continue. Initial radiographs may be negative, and bone-scan or MRI studies may be required for diagnosis. After 3 to 4 weeks, a thin sclerotic line may be visible on plain radiographs. Treatment includes immobilization, ice, NSAIDs, and non–weight bearing.

Plantar Fascial Tear

Plantar fascial tear is rare because the plantar fascia is thick, tough, and resilient to pressure and trauma. Patients present with a history of trauma, a feeling of sharp pain, often accompanied by a pop or a tearing sensation in the plantar heel or arch area. There is a correlation between previous multiple corticosteroid injections and plantar fascial tear. Presentation includes swelling and often ecchymosis. A palpable defect in the fascia may be present. Confirmation by MRI may be necessary, although plantar fascial tear is often a clinical diagnosis. Treatment includes immobilization, rest, ice, NSAIDs, and non–weight bearing with crutches, often for a period of 4 to 6 weeks.[11]

Tarsal Tunnel Syndrome

Tarsal tunnel presents with a history of paresthesia, and pain to the heel. The posterior tibial nerve passes under the laciniate ligament accompanied by the posterior tibial artery and veins. It branches into the medial plantar nerve, lateral plantar nerve, and the medial calcaneal nerve. Compression occurs due to trauma, varicosities of the vena comicantes, or hypertrophy of the ligament. Presentation may include pain in the area of the port-au-pedis or directly inferior to the plantar calcaneal tuberosity. The Tinel test is performed by percussing the tarsal tunnel and eliciting pain or tingling sensation distally. The Veilleux test is performed by percussing the tarsal tunnel and eliciting the pain and tingling sensation proximally and distally. Nerve conduction velocity test and distal latency studies are necessary to establish the diagnosis. Treatment includes injection therapy, oral medication, or nerve decompression through surgery.

Medial Calcaneal Nerve Entrapment

The medial calcaneal nerve arises off the posterior tibial nerve, usually distal to the laciniate ligament. In some cases, branching may occur more proximally. The nerve courses plantarly beneath the heel and serves the medial, plantar, and lateral aspects of the heel. Entrapment may occur as a result of pressure because the nerve passes underneath the calcaneal tuberosity. Symptoms are more neurologic and include paresthesia, tingling, and burning. Treatment includes reducing pressure on the nerve through surgical decompression and injection therapy to reduce fibrosis.

Plantar Calcaneal Bursitis

The plantar calcaneal bursa may become inflamed with weight bearing or prolonged trauma. Symptoms may mimic those of plantar fasciitis, with pain on direct compression of the plantar calcaneal tuberosity. There may be mild edema but no ecchymosis. Radiographs will be negative and this condition usually responds well to off-loading and injection therapy.

Bone Contusion

A bone contusion occurs with trauma to the calcaneus. Often the patient presents after a minor injury, such as slipping on a stair and jamming the heel into the floor. Radiographs are negative and there may be no ecchymosis or edema. There is pain to compression of the plantar heel, with no history of poststatic dyskinesia. Treatment is usually symptomatic with ice, NSAIDs, and off-loading.

DIAGNOSTIC TESTING

Generally the diagnosis of plantar fasciitis is clinical, based on the history of pain, poststatic dyskinesia, absence of trauma, and edema along with the physical examination.

Radiographs

Radiographs are the most common diagnostic test performed for heel pain and plantar fasciitis. Because plantar fasciitis and heel spur syndrome are closely related, lateral, medial oblique, and lateral oblique radiographs of the foot can confirm the presence of a plantar calcaneal spur (**Fig. 1**). A heel spur may be present, but these have also been reported to be present in 27% of people without any symptoms. Radiographs can also confirm later-stage stress fracture, bone tumors, bone cysts, periostitis, and erosions due to infection or rheumatologic causes.

Diagnostic Ultrasound

Normal plantar fascia is hyperechoic and isoechoic with adjacent fat. On the sagittal plane, the fascia is recognized by its striated appearance secondary to the orientation of the fibers.[12] In patients with clinical symptoms of plantar fasciitis, the proximal end of

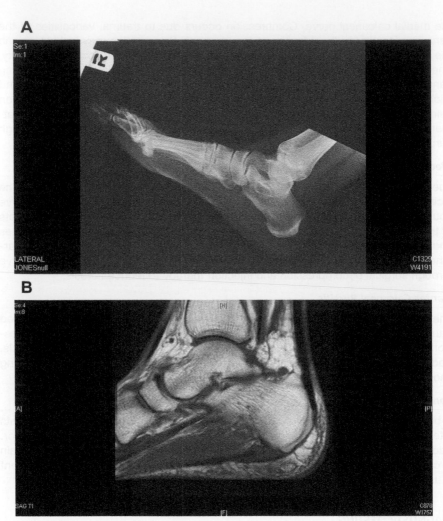

Fig. 1. (*A, B*) Heel spur noted plantarly.

the fascia is hypoechoic, which can be seen clearly when compared with the surrounding soft tissue. Plantar fascia is also significantly thicker in patients with plantar fasciitis. Symptomatic patients were seen to have fascia measuring 4 mm or more in thickness, whereas those of asymptomatic patients measured 4 mm or less.[2,12]

MRI

MRI is not usually used to diagnose plantar fasciitis. However, it is a useful tool to differentiate between the various causes of heel pain. Most commonly seen is perifascial edema, which appears as poorly circumscribed areas of high signal intensity on the short-tau inversion recovery (STIR) images in the soft tissues superficial or deep to the plantar fascia.[13] The second most common finding is bone marrow edema of the calcaneus at the insertion of the plantar fascia. The area of the edema is small. This may also be seen when trauma has occurred to the heel. The third most common findings is high signal intensity within the plantar fascia on T2 and STIR images that may show some degree of fascial tear. On T1-weighted spin-echo MRI, intermediate signal intensity within the plantar fascia can be seen as well as aponeurotic thickening greater than 5 mm on T1 sequences.

Computerized Tomography Scan

Computerized tomography (CT) scan be performed if calcaneal stress fracture is suspected. Generally, MRI or CT would be considered only in those cases recalcitrant to treatment and for those patients with a high index of suspicion for the other causes of heel pain.

Technetium 99 Bone Scan

A bone scan is often positive with chronic heel pain and plantar fasciitis due to chronic periostitis and inflammation, with increased activity in the periosteum. A technetium 99 bone scan can also diagnose fatigue or a stress fracture. There will be diffuse, intense increased activity with a stress fracture, whereas plantar fasciitis will show focal uptake in the area of the medial calcaneal tuberosity.

Nerve Conduction Velocity and Electromyography Test

Distal latencies are performed if tarsal tunnel is suspected. Normal distal latencies are 4.1 and 4.7 milliseconds for the medial and lateral plantar nerves, respectively. Patients with tarsal tunnel syndrome show delays in the distal latency studies. However, In some cases of tarsal tunnel these studies may be normal.

CONSERVATIVE TREATMENT OPTIONS
Low Dye Strapping

Low dye strapping is often an effective treatment modality in mild to moderate cases. The strapping uses adhesive tape to immobilize the foot and decreases the distance between the origin and insertion of the plantar fascia, thus relieving plantar strain. Tape will loosen in time, often quickly, and may prove less effective in severe cases. Relief with plantar support via strapping often gives a good indication of the efficacy of orthotics in a particular patient.[14]

Footwear

The American Academy of Podiatric Sports Medicine advocates a minimum 2.5-cm (1-inch) heel height with a strong stable midfoot shank and relatively uninhibited forefoot flexibility for treatment of plantar fasciitis. Going barefoot and wearing sandals are not recommended.

Stretching of the Achilles Tendon and Plantar Fascia

Porter and colleagues[15] studied 94 patients with plantar fasciitis on a program of stretching of the Achilles tendon. The patients were separated into 2 groups. Group 1 stretched 3 times per day for 3 minutes each session. Group 2 stretched twice each day for five 20-second periods each session. Each groups stretched for a period of 4 months. The investigators noted improvement in foot and ankle function for both groups, with no significant differences between group 1 and group 2. Most physicians today incorporate a vigorous program of stretching in patients with plantar fasciitis.[16]

DiGiovanni and colleagues[17] compared protocols of Achilles tendon stretching versus specific stretching of the plantar fascia. With the plantar fascia stretch, the affected side is placed on the contralateral knee, the ankle is held dorsiflexed, and the toes are moved into dorsiflexion by hand. This exercise causes stretch and tension in the plantar fascia. Improvement was found at 8 weeks in 52% of patients, compared with 22% in the Achilles tendon–only stretching program.

Night Splints

Night splints are worn to keep the ankle in neutral to slightly dorsiflexed position. This technique prevents contracture of the plantar fascia while resting at night and promotes stretching of the Achilles tendon. Batt and colleagues[18] evaluated 33 patients with plantar fasciitis for the effectiveness of ankle dorsiflexion night splints. Seventeen patients were in the treatment group, and 16 were controls. All 17 patients in this study experienced substantial relief, with an average time to resolution of 12.5 weeks. Patients often complain that the splints are uncomfortable for the first few nights, but the discomfort generally becomes less in time.

Physical Therapy

Physical therapy treatments have been one of the cornerstones of plantar fasciitis, although studies show pain relief in patients after 2 weeks but no statistically significant relief after 1 month.[19] Ice is prescribed each night to decrease edema and inflammation. Other modalities, such as whirlpool and ultrasound treatments, are performed 3 times per week for 3 to 4 weeks as part of the physical therapy regimen.[20] They are combined with passive stretching of the tendoachilles and plantar fascia.

Antiinflammatory Agents/Oral Corticosteroids

Antiinflammatory agents have been widely used in the treatment of plantar fasciitis, whether they are given orally, topically, or via injection. NSAIDs are given to decrease inflammation but care must be taken in patients with gastritis or ulcer disease, renal disease, or reflux esophagitis. They are best used as short-term therapy. New topical antiinflammatory agents, such as diclofenac sodium gel, can be used, but studies on efficacy have been limited. The gel is applied directly to intact skin around the location of the pain.

Injection of Corticosteroid

Care must be taken with injections so that atrophy of the soft tissue does not occur. Gill[21] advises injecting deep to the plantar fascia, between the fascia and the calcaneus, to avoid atrophy and necrosis of the calcaneal fat pad. Generally, corticosteroid injections are given in a series of 3, spaced a few weeks apart.

Crawford and colleagues[22] concluded that pain scores were reduced after corticosteroid injection, and remained so after 1 month, with maximum benefit for 6 to 8 weeks. However, at the 3- and 6-month marks, no significant differences were noted.

Complications of injections include rupture of plantar fascia. Acevedo and Beskin[23] reported that, in a group of 765 patients with a clinical diagnosis of plantar fasciitis, 51 were diagnosed with a plantar fascial rupture. Of these ruptures, 44 (86%) were associated with prior corticosteroid injection.[23] Balasubramanian and Prathap[24] believed that local steroid injections cause focal necrosis of collagenous tissue and can predispose ruptures of tendon or fascia.

Orthoses

Scherer[25] stated that the most important part of orthotic success was to mechanically control the midtarsal joint. Lynch and colleagues[26] carried out a prospective study comparing the success of orthoses with NSAIDs and steroid injections. Orthotics had an 80% success rate, compared with 33% and 30% success rates with NSAIDs and steroid injections respectively.

Extracorporeal Shock-Wave Therapy

In 2000, the Food and Drug Administration approved the use of extracorporeal shock-wave (ESWT) therapy to treat plantar fasciitis. Sound waves are propagated to damaged tissues to induce microtrauma. This microtrauma stimulates healing by attracting blood vessels and nutrients to the plantar fascia. ESWT comes in low waves and high waves. Waves are considered low energy if the flux density ranges from 0.05 to 0.10 mL/mm^2 making local anesthetics unnecessary. Side effects consist of redness at the area of therapy, pain, and swelling.

Through an acoustic lens, the focus of the shock-wave source, or heel spur, is centered with the c-arm. This focus should cover an area of 50 mm in the axis of the shock wave and a diameter of 7.0 mm perpendicular to the shock-wave axis. The shock-wave unit is placed on the foot along the medial aspect of the heel over a layer of ultrasound gel.

Rompe and colleagues[27] studied 112 patients who received 3 treatments of 1000 impulses weekly or 3 treatments of 10 impulses weekly. These patients were evaluated on the visual analog scale to assess pain on palpation, ambulation, and pain at rest/night after 6 months of treatment and 5 years after treatment. Patients were instructed to stop all therapy for 6 weeks before the extracorporeal shock-wave therapy. After 6 months and 5 years, the group who received the treatments of 1000 impulses showed significantly less pain on palpation, ambulation, and after rest or at night compared with the group who only received 10 impulses for 3 weeks.

In another double-blind randomized study, Haake and colleagues[28] compared ESWT with a placebo in 272 patients. All patients had suffered from chronic plantar fasciitis for more than 6 months. The ESWT group received 4000 impulses of positive energy flux density (0.08 mJ/mm^2) under local anesthesia every 2 weeks for 12 weeks. The placebo group received therapy consisting of a polyethylene foil filled with air, also under local anesthesia. Final results between the 2 groups revealed no significant difference in pain level, ambulation, or need for additional therapy at the end of the 12 weeks and after 1-year follow-up. A similar study by Buchbinder and colleagues[29] confirmed no statistically significant difference between the ESWT group and placebo.

SURGICAL TREATMENT OPTIONS

When conservative management fails, which occurs in approximately 10% of patients, surgical options should be considered. Symptoms should be present for more than 6 months before surgery should be discussed.

Open Plantar Fasciotomy

Open plantar fasciotomy allows for release of the tight plantar fascial bands. An incision is made along the anterior medial aspect of the heel distal to the insertion of the plantar fascia. Once the soft tissue is freed from the fascia, the medial bands are transected. If a heel spur is present, a rasp may be used to smooth down the prominence. Some surgeons will free the abductor hallucis muscle to prevent nerve entrapment from occurring. Open surgery has risks; approximately 25% of patients will still experience heel pain after the surgery.[30] Over-release of the plantar fascia may lead to flat-foot complications. Nerve entrapments can occur, as well as pain along the scar.

Contompasis[31] performed a 3-year retrospective study of 126 surgeries for plantar fasciitis. Plantar fascial release provided 36% satisfactory relief.[31] A combination of fascial release and spur resection allowed 44.3% to have complete resolution of pain and 45.2% to have improvement in pain, whereas 10.5% had no relief.

Endoscopic Plantar Fasciotomy

Endoscopic plantar fasciotomy (EPF) has become more popular because of its minimally invasive nature and visualization of the fascia. It minimizes complications and recovery time compared with open procedures. EPF is performed by creating a small incision along the medial aspect of the heel at the anteriomedial border of the calcaneus. Blunt dissection separates the subcutaneous fat from the fascia inferiorly and superiorly. A cannula with a trochar is then passed from medial to lateral. Some surgeons choose to make a second incision along the lateral aspect of the heel at the tip of the trochar. Others choose to use only 1 portal for the entire procedure. At this point the endoscope and the cutting device are inserted. The superficial and deep layers of the medial band of the plantar fascia are then transected to the point where the medial band ends, which is approximately halfway across the fascia.[32] Satisfaction ranged from 60% to 80% with this procedure in relief of heel pain. Complications after endoscopic plantar fasciotomies include heel pain, calcaneal stress fractures, lateral column pain, incisional pain, nerve entrapment, and postoperative infection.

Cryosurgery

Percutaneous cryosurgery uses subfreezing temperatures to produce analgesic effects. The areas of maximum tenderness are marked on the foot. A stab incision is made along the anterior medial aspect of the heel. A probe is used to bluntly dissect the subcutaneous tissue from the plantar fascia. The cryostar plantar fascial probe is then inserted inferior to the plantar fascia up to the point marked on the foot. A nerve sensor in the probe determines the course of the nerves in the fascia. Three minutes of cryosurgery are performed, followed by 30 seconds of thawing. Another course of 3 minutes of cryosurgery is then performed. It is important to explain to the patient that numbness will occur to the plantar heel for many months after the procedure. In a study by Cavazos and colleagues,[33] out of 137 feet, 77.4% of the patients were considered to be successes after cryosurgery. This procedure is still being studied for the effects on nerve and soft tissue after the freeze-thaw cycles.

Radiofrequency Nerve Ablation

Radiofrequency ablation is another minimally invasive procedure that ablates the nerve by generating a 5-mm sphere of heat around the tip of the electrode. The point of maximum tenderness is marked on the foot. A 22-gauge insulated needle is inserted into the marked location and an electrode is inserted to stimulate the nerves. If fasciculation is noted, the motor nerve is being stimulated and the needle needs to be pulled back until a purely sensory nerve is being stimulated. At this point, the generator is increased to 90°C for 90 seconds. Patients are allowed to bear weight immediately after the procedure. Liden and colleagues[34] performed a retrospective study on 31 feet that received radiofrequency ablation therapy to the heel. The mean visual analog pain score was 8.12 before treatment, and 2.07 at 6 months. Complications include hematoma at the site of entry from the cannula.

Coblation Therapy

Coblation therapy with Topaz is a form of bipolar radiofrequency. It causes microscopic damage to the fascia, which increases the blood supply to the fascia, bringing healing factors, and breaks up the nocioceptors. It requires a small stab incision at the medial aspect of the heel to allow for insertion of the cannula and obturator. The Topaz wand should be connected to a saline solution and placed on the surface of the fascia.

It allows for 0.5 seconds of pressure, creating perforations at 5-mm intervals with 1-, 3-, and 5-mm depths. The patient is immobilized for 3 weeks and then returned to ambulatory status.

SUMMARY

Plantar fasciitis is a common cause of heel pain. Once clinically diagnosed, the rehabilitation time through conservative or surgical management may last for many months.

REFERENCES

1. Riddle DL, Pulisic M, Pidcoe P, et al. Risk factors for plantar fasciitis: a matched case-control study. J Bone Joint Surg Am 2003;85:872–7.
2. Berkowitz JF, Kier R, Rudicel S. Plantar fasciitis: MR imaging. Radiology 1991; 179:665–7.
3. Myerson MIn: Foot and ankle disorders, vol. 2. Philadelphia: WB Saunders; 2000. 837–40.
4. Lemont H, Ammirati KM, Usen N. Plantar fasciitis: a degenerative process (Fasciosis) without inflammation. J Am Podiatr Med Assoc 2003;93(3):234–7.
5. Wearing SC, Smeathers JE, Urry SR, et al. The pathomechanics of plantar fasciitis. Sports Med 2006;36(7):585–611.
6. Hicks JH. The foot as a support. Acta Anat 1955;25:34–5.
7. Salathe EP. A biomechanical model of the foot. J Biomech 1986;19:980–100 l.
8. Carpenter JE, Flanagan CL, Thomopoulos S, et al. The effects of overuse combined with intrinsic or extrinsic alterations in an animal model of rotator cuff tendinosis. Am J Sports Med 1998;26:801–7.
9. Prichasuk S. The relationship of pes planus and calcaneal spur to plantar heel pain. Clin Orthop 1994;306:192–6.
10. McCarty DJ. Arthritis and allied conditions. 9th edition. Philadelphia: Lea and Febiger; 1979. p. 470–2, 602–3, 617–8, 638.
11. Saxena A, Fullem B. Plantar fascia ruptures in athletes. Am J Sports Med 2004; 32:662–5.
12. Gibbon WW, Long G. Ultrasound of the plantar aponeurosis (fascia). Skeletal Radiol 1999;28:21–6.
13. Grasel RP, Schweitzer ME, Kovalovich AM. MR imaging of plantar fasciitis: edema, tears, and occult marrow abnormalities correlated with outcome. AJR Am J Roentgenol 1999;173:699–701.
14. Yale I. Podiatric medicine. Baltimore: Williams and Wilkins; 1974. p. 219–20.
15. Porter D, Barrill E, Oneacre K, et al. The effects of duration and frequency of Achilles tendon stretching on dorsiflexion and outcome in painful heel syndrome: a randomized, blinded, control study. Foot Ankle Int 2002;23:619–24.
16. League AC. Current concepts review. Foot Ankle Int 2008;29:360.
17. DiGiovanni BF, Nawoczenski DA, Malay DP, et al. Plantar fascia-specific stretching exercise improves outcomes in patients with chronic plantar fasciitis. J Bone Joint Surg Am 2006;88:1775–81.
18. Batt ME, Tanji JL, Skattim N, et al. Plantar fasciitis: a prospective randomized clinical trial of the tension night splint. Foot Ankle Int 1999;6:158–62.
19. Leach RE, Seavey MS, Salter DK. Results of surgery in athletes with plantar fasciitis. Foot Ankle 1986;7:156–61.
20. Gudeman SD, Eisele SA, Heidt RS, et al. Treatment of plantar fasciitis by iontophoresis of 0.4% dexamethasone: a randomized, double-blind placebo-controlled study. Am J Sports Med 1997;25:312–6.

21. Gill LH. Plantar fasciitis: diagnosis and conservative management. Am Acad Orthop Surg 1997;5:109–17.
22. Crawford F, Atkins D, Young P, et al. Steroid injections for heel pain: evidence of short-term effectiveness. A randomized controlled trial. Rheumatology 1999;38: 974–7.
23. Acevedo JI, Beskin JL. Complications of plantar fascia ruptures associated with corticosteroid injections. Foot Ankle Int 1998;19(2):91–7.
24. Balasubramaniam P, Prathap K. The effect of injection of hydrocortisone into rabbit calcaneal tendons. J Bone Joint Surg Br 1972;54(4):729–34.
25. Scherer PR. Heel spur syndrome. pathomechanics and nonsurgical treatment. J Am Pod Med Assoc 1991;81:68–72.
26. Lynch DM, Goforth WP, Martin JE, et al. Conservative treatment of plantar fasciitis. A prospective study. J Am Podiatr Med Assoc 1998;88(8):375–80.
27. Rompe JD, Schoellner C, Bernhard NE. Evaluation of low-energy extracorporeal shock-wave application for treatment of chronic plantar fasciitis. J Bone Joint Surg Am 2002;84:335–41.
28. Haake M, Buch M, Schoellner C, et al. Extracorporeal shock wave therapy for plantar fasciitis: randomised controlled multicentre trial. Br Med J 2003;327:75–9.
29. Buchbinder R, Ptasznik R, Gordon J, et al. Ultrasound-guided extracorporeal shock wave therapy for plantar fasciitis: a randomized controlled trial. J Am Med Assoc 2002;288:1364–72.
30. Buchbinder R. Clinical practice: plantar fasciitis. N Engl J Med 2004;350: 2159–66.
31. Contompasis JP. Surgical treatment of calcaneal spurs: a three-year postsurgical study. J Am Podiatr Med Assoc 1974;64(12):987–99.
32. Hogan KA, Webb D, Shereff M. Endoscopic plantar fascia release. Foot Ankle Int 2004;25(12):875–81.
33. Cavazos J, Khan KH, D'Antoni AV, et al. Cryosurgery for the treatment of heel pain. Foot Ankle Int 2009;53(6):500–5.
34. Liden B, Simmons M, Landsman AS. A retrospective analysis of 22 patients treated with percutaneous radiofrequency nerve ablation for prolonged moderate to severe heel pain associated with plantar fasciitis. J Foot Ankle Surg 2009; 48(6):642–7.

Internal and External Fixation Approaches to the Surgical Management of Calcaneal Fractures

John J. Stapleton, DPM[a,b,]*, Gennady Kolodenker, DPM[c], Thomas Zgonis, DPM[d]

KEYWORDS

- Calcaneal fractures • Open reduction • External fixation
- Foot • Complications

Displaced intraarticular fractures of the calcaneus are usually the result of high-energy trauma and are commonly encountered with falls from a significant height or high-speed motor vehicle accidents.[1–5] The initial evaluation, which is commonly performed by the emergency room physicians or trauma service, is performed to thoroughly evaluate patients for multiple traumatic injuries that can occur with high-energy trauma. A thorough evaluation should be performed on the rest of the musculoskeletal system, and the head, chest, and abdomen. Common contiguous fractures associated with fractures of the calcaneus involve the spine, contralateral lower extremity, and the wrist.[6–8]

A lower-extremity vascular assessment needs always to be performed for the presence of a palpable dorsalis pedis and posterior tibial artery. Doppler studies or angiography may be obtained if needed. Arterial injury, although rare, can be associated with high-energy trauma and especially with open and displaced fractures of the medial wall of the calcaneus. In cases of severe peripheral vascular disease that is commonly found in smokers and patients with diabetes mellitus, open reduction and internal fixation (ORIF) of calcaneal fractures is contraindicated.

---

[a] Foot and Ankle Surgery, VSAS Orthopaedics; Allentown, PA, USA
[b] Penn State College of Medicine, Hershey, PA, USA
[c] University Hospital, University of Medicine and Dentistry of New Jersey, 150 Bergen Street, Newark, NJ, USA
[d] Division of Podiatric Medicine and Surgery, Department of Orthopaedic Surgery, The University of Texas Health Science Center at San Antonio, 7703 Floyd Curl Drive–MSC 7776, San Antonio, TX 78229, USA
* Corresponding author. Foot and Ankle Surgery, VSAS Orthopaedics, Allentown, PA.
E-mail address: jostaple@hotmail.com

Clin Podiatr Med Surg 27 (2010) 381–392
doi:10.1016/j.cpm.2010.03.003
0891-8422/10/$ – see front matter © 2010 Published by Elsevier Inc.

podiatric.theclinics.com

A detailed neurologic lower-extremity examination of the plantar aspect of the foot also needs to be performed in responsive patients because the tibial nerve can be injured at the time of calcaneal fracture displacement. Other times, the patients report intact plantar sensation initially with altered or incomplete sensory loss postoperatively. Patients with calcaneal fractures are often in severe pain and the examination might be a challenge for the clinician to determine if incomplete sensory loss was apparent initially. Compartment syndrome as a result of increased pressures within the subcalcaneal and foot compartments may be present and also need to be monitored and addressed if clinically suspected. Compartment syndrome can also alter sensation. A high index of suspicion is necessary.

Inspection of the soft-tissue envelope is paramount for closed calcaneal fractures in which an anticipated ORIF is planned. The soft tissues must be assessed for fracture blisters, superficial and deep abrasions, and the degree of soft-tissue swelling. Surgery may need to be delayed until the associated soft-tissue swelling has dissipated to the point that a positive pinch test or skin wrinkles are apparent.

Plain radiographic evaluation includes lateral, anteroposterior, and oblique views of the foot, an anteroposterior view of the ankle, and a long axial view of the calcaneus. The anteroposterior and oblique foot views are evaluated to determine the presence or extent of intraarticular involvement of the calcaneal cuboid joint. The lateral view of the hindfoot determines the presence of joint depression or tongue type fractures. A decrease in Bohler's angle, an increase in the angle of Gissane, and a double density sign on the lateral radiograph are indicative of an intraarticular joint depression of the subtalar joint. Tongue type fractures exit through the posterior superior aspect of the calcaneal tuberosity. The axial view of the calcaneus determines the position of the calcaneal tuberosity in relation to the primary fracture line, evaluates for any fractures of the sustentaculum tali, and also displays the degree of the calcaneal widening. Often, the calcaneal tuberosity is in a varus position but a valgus rotation, although rare, may be present. The anteroposterior view of the ankle is useful in severely pulverized calcaneal fractures that may be associated with dislocation or an ankle fracture. In addition, fleck or rim fractures off the distal fibula may be indicative of associated peroneal tendon dislocation.

CT is indicated if intraarticular calcaneal involvement is present or suspected. Often, intraarticular fractures are missed when the fracture line extends into the lateral aspect of the subtalar joint. As a result, the large medial fracture fragment and sustentaculum tali are not depressed, which results in normal-appearing Bohler's and Gissane's angles on the initial lateral radiograph. Often, the double density sign on the initial lateral radiograph is the only indication of this fracture pattern. Given the anatomic complexity of calcaneal fractures it is the authors' preference to obtain a CT scan on almost every calcaneal fracture to exclude the possibility of intraarticular involvement in equivocal cases and to serve as a preoperative planning tool in obvious intraarticular calcaneal fractures.

CT images should be obtained in 2 mm intervals in the axial, sagittal, and 30-degree semi-coronal planes. The coronal views should be perpendicular to the posterior facet of the subtalar joint and the axial views should be parallel to the foot to avoid distortion of the reconstruction images. CT images with three-dimensional (3-D) reconstructive views may be required for preoperative planning in complex scenarios if a 3-D picture cannot be pieced together after evaluating all the CT images.[9] Understanding the pathoanatomy of each calcaneal fracture through CT imaging is paramount to obtaining an anatomic surgical reduction.

The axial CT images are evaluated for fracture lines involving the anterior process and floor of the sinus tarsi. Often, the axial images are too incomplete to evaluate

the posterior facet of the subtalar joint. The semi-coronal CT images are used to evaluate the articular fracture fragments of the middle and posterior facets of the subtalar
joint. The semi-coronal view is also used to classify the fracture and to further determine if surgical reconstruction or a primary subtalar joint arthrodesis should be performed. Four or more fracture fragments of the subtalar joint are treated with
primary subtalar joint arthrodesis as poor surgical outcomes are evident with attempted ORIF.[2] In addition, the semi-coronal views are beneficial to determine the position
of the tuberosity fragment in relation to the primary fracture line, evaluate the displacement of the medial wall of the calcaneus, and to determine the degree of lateral calcaneal wall expansion. The sagittal reconstruction views assist in obtaining a 3-D picture
of the calcaneal fracture and also determine the placement of impacted intraarticular
fracture fragments. Delineation between tongue type and joint depressed fracture
fragments are also determined. Despite the advantages of CT imaging, evaluation
of the fracture pattern alone cannot definitively determine which fractures should be
surgically repaired and by what method. The overall method of treatment is dependent
on the fracture pattern, soft-tissue envelope, other contiguous fractures, and systemic
medical conditions.

The initial treatment of closed calcaneal fractures usually consists of strict elevation
of the affected lower extremity and a Jones compression dressing. Calcaneal fractures are notorious for significant edema and hematoma formation and ORIF is usually
delayed to further evaluate the soft-tissue envelope and to appreciate the soft-tissue
injury before proceeding with surgery. An exception to this approach is when a fracture
fragment produces pressure on the skin that will most likely lead to skin necrosis,
which has to be addressed promptly. These fracture fragments are usually seen in
severely displaced tongue type fractures, avulsion fractures of the posterior superior
calcaneal tuberosity, and calcaneal dislocations. Full resolution of soft-tissue edema
may require about 3 weeks or even more in some cases. In these case scenarios,
ORIF may not be amenable through an extensile lateral approach, and often fracture
reduction may need to be considered with minimally invasive techniques, such as
limited combined open reduction with internal and external fixation techniques. These
minimally invasive techniques may not achieve perfect anatomic reduction but are
used to restore the alignment of the tuberosity, improve the heel height and width,
and better align the calcaneus for a staged, subtalar joint fusion if needed.

OPEN CALCANEAL FRACTURES

The initial presentation of an open calcaneal fractures is usually staged in reconstruction and overall management. This management includes a thorough irrigation and
debridement of the wound that needs to be performed within the first 6 to 8 hours,
the golden period of the injury, if feasible. A one-touch rule should be instituted
between the trauma and medical teams to minimize further wound contamination,
because further exploration and handling of the open fracture needs to be performed
in the operating room.

A combination of intravenous antibiotics and meticulous debridement and copious
amounts of saline irrigation are instituted at the initial surgery. This initial stage should
include reduction or repositioning of fracture fragments through the open fracture to
avoid tension and skin necrosis. At times, the use of external fixation or temporary
placement of Steinman pins may be required to facilitate wound closure and to
prevent further wound necrosis until a more definitive procedure can be performed.
The goal in this initial stage is not to necessarily achieve anatomic reduction but to
achieve fracture stabilization by preventing further soft-tissue compromise and

eventual skin necrosis. Once the wound can be closed primarily, the fracture is commonly treated in the same manner as a closed calcaneal fracture. Open fractures that are not amenable to primary skin closure are further treated with splint or cast immobilization, limited open reduction techniques, or external fixation (**Fig. 1**).

NONOPERATIVE MANAGEMENT

Calcaneal fractures that are non-displaced or with less than 2 mm of intraarticular displacement can be treated conservatively. Often, non-displaced calcaneal fractures must be radiographically re-evaluated during the first 2 to 4 weeks to exclude later displacement. Patients need to be immobilized with strict non-weight–bearing status with all non-displaced intraarticular fractures. The major fracture lines extending into the joint must be completely healed before initiating a weight-bearing status. The time frame ranges from 6 to 12 weeks depending on the degree of comminution within the body and the potential for collapse. In addition, intraarticular fractures of the calcaneus that are non-displaced still display significant comminution within the body of the calcaneus. At times, a repeat CT scan may be required initially and repeated later to confirm interval healing and to be certain bone voids inferior to the joint are not evident, which could lead to later collapse, malunion, and joint incongruity as patients progress to weight-bearing status. Extra-articular fractures involving the inferior aspect of the tuberosity or anterior process may be treated initially with a protective offloading device and further progressive weight bearing as tolerated by the patients.

EXTENSILE LATERAL INCISION FOR OPEN REDUCTION AND INTERNAL FIXATION

The extensile lateral incision has become the standard approach to performing ORIF of displaced joint depressed calcaneal fractures.[10] Advantages to this incisional approach include the direct anatomic reduction of the posterior facet while reconstructing the entire calcaneal body (**Fig. 2**). In addition, the peroneal tendons can be inspected for subluxation and repaired if required.

Patients are either positioned in the lateral decubitus or prone position on a radiolucent fracture table to facilitate exposure and to allow for adequate intraoperative fluoroscopic imaging. The extensile lateral incision has had few modifications over the recent years to prevent flap necrosis and wound healing complications. It is based on creating a full thickness flap that includes the periosteum of the lateral calcaneus, sural nerve, transected calcaneal fibular ligament, and peroneal tendons. The vertical arm of the incision is made just lateral and anterior to the Achilles tendon and posterior to the sural nerve and lateral calcaneal artery. The horizontal arm of the incision is made at the junction of the plantar heel pad and the lateral skin. Fashioning the incision in this manner avoids injury to major angiosomes of the lateral foot and ankle including the lateral calcaneal artery and branch of the peroneal artery. Additional collateral flow to the full-thickness flap is supplied by the lateral malleolar and lateral tarsal artery.

The flap is retracted by placing 0.062 in smooth Kirchner wires into the fibula, neck of the talus, and cuboid to facilitate retraction while avoiding any further handling of the flap. Fracture reduction begins with removing the lateral wall and placing this piece in normal saline followed by inserting a 4 mm partially threaded half pin into the calcaneal tuberosity fracture fragment. In joint depressed calcaneal fractures, the half pin is placed from lateral to medial in the inferior portion of the calcaneal tuberosity. In tongue type fractures, the half pin is typically placed from posterior to anterior in the superior aspect of the calcaneal tuberosity. The half pin is then used as a joy stick to place longitudinal traction and a varus force initially to dislodge and identify the superior lateral fracture fragment of the posterior facet of the subtalar joint. This

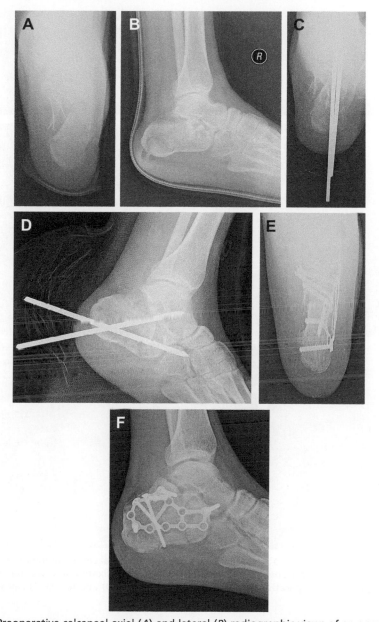

Fig. 1. Preoperative calcaneal axial (*A*) and lateral (*B*) radiographic views of an open calcaneal fracture medially and a significant varus rotation. Patient was brought to the operating room immediately for a meticulous wound debridement and irrigation and further stabilization of the fracture fragments with two Steinmann pins (*C, D*). Patient was eventually brought back to the operating room for removal of the temporarily fixation followed by standard open reduction and internal fixation. Final postoperative views at 6 months (*E, F*).

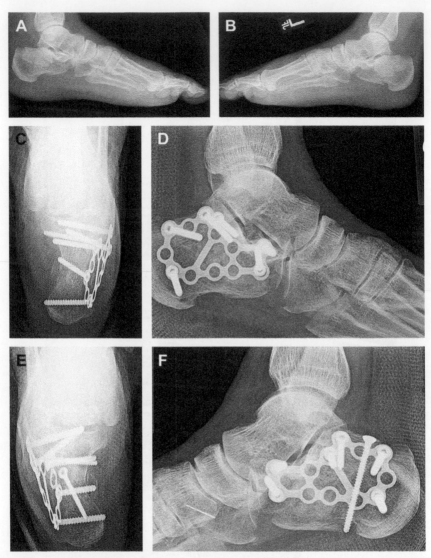

Fig. 2. Preoperative lateral radiographic views (A, B) of bilateral calcaneal fractures. Patient underwent a bilateral calcaneal fracture repair with internal fixation and via the extensile lateral approach. Postoperative radiographs of the right (C, D) and left (E, F) calcaneus at 4 months.

fracture fragment can be removed and preserved in saline to facilitate visualization of the primary fracture line and the medial wall. The medial wall is then reduced while longitudinal traction is placed on the half pin along with a medial force and a valgus tilt. A curved elevator can be inserted under the constant medial fracture fragment to facilitate reduction. The reduction is held provisionally with at least two 1.6 mm Steinmann pins. Reduction of the medial wall is then confirmed under fluoroscopic axial images. At this time, the floor of the sinus tarsi and the anterior process fracture fragments are reduced and held with provisional Steinman pins. The posterior facet is then anatomically positioned starting with the medial most fracture fragments first because these are stabilized with Steinmann pins. The superior lateral fracture fragment is then positioned and held with at least two 1.6 mm Steinman pins while lag screw fixation is achieved. Joint reduction is confirmed under direct visualization and by confirming alignment through a lateral and Broden's view under fluoroscopic imaging.

The bone defect below the posterior facet of the subtalar joint and throughout the calcaneal body is then typically packed with allogenic bone graft and the lateral wall is then placed back into position followed by the application of a calcaneal plate. Various calcaneal plates exist each with their own design and proposed advantages. Calcaneal plates that offer optional locking screws have recently gained popularity among various orthopedic industries. However, the literature does not support any superior clinical benefit in using locking plates versus non-locking plates in the surgical management of calcaneal fractures. In addition, locking plates have a thicker profile and often give the surgeon a false sense of achieving stable fixation. It is the authors' preference to use non-locking plates to achieve osseous fixation unless severe osteoporosis or comminution is present. Screw configuration should be meticulously planned in anatomic placement and orientation to achieve bicortical screw purchase. The surgeon needs to be aware of the anatomic locations of the calcaneus that is associated with dense subchondral and cortical bone. These regions include the immediate inferior aspect of the posterior facet of the subtalar joint, the area just proximal to the calcaneal-cuboid joint, and the subcortical bone located around the perimeter of the calcaneal tuberosity. In addition, the goal of ORIF is not to place as many screws as possible but to achieve anatomic reduction. Often, the body of the calcaneus displays severe comminution and after fracture reduction a bone void is usually present. This region of the calcaneus is often not amendable to screw fixation and locking screws placed in this region are not advantageous in providing further osseous stability. Prior to wound closure, the peroneal tendons can be examined for subluxation. If subluxation is present a separate 3-cm incision is made after the flap is closed by anchoring the peroneal tendon sheath to the fibula either through small drill holes within the posterior lateral rim of the distal fibula or by placing bone anchors. The goal of the repair is to eliminate this false pouch to prevent further peroneal tendon subluxation. Closure of the flap is typically closed in two layers. Patients are then placed into a well-padded Jones compression dressing and non-weight–bearing posterior splint with the foot held in a neutral or slightly dorsiflexed position.

PRIMARY SUBTALAR JOINT FUSION

A primary subtalar joint fusion is indicated for calcaneal fractures that involve four-part (or more) fractures of the posterior facet of the subtalar joint. Sanders and colleagues[2] reported the poor outcomes that were evident after ORIF of this subtype of intraarticular calcaneal fractures and advocated primary fusion as the alternative. At times, two- and three-part fractures may be well reduced but the chondral injury sustained would likely result in posttraumatic arthritis.[2,11] The management of these fracture patterns is not well established and the literature remains controversial. Other surgical dilemmas arise when an ORIF cannot be performed secondarily to poor soft-tissue envelope, open fracture, and resolution of soft-tissue edema that has taken longer than 3 to 4 weeks. These case scenarios are typically best managed with a primary subtalar joint fusion. Calcaneal fractures present in patients who are diabetic with peripheral neuropathy are at times best managed with a primary subtalar joint fusion.

In addition, patients who are diabetic with multiple comorbidities and dense peripheral neuropathy, previous Charcot deformity, morbid obesity, and contralateral lower extremity amputation may be better suited with a stable subtalar joint fusion as opposed to an attempted ORIF (**Fig. 3**). Some of the advantages to performing a primary subtalar joint fusion within this patient population include the use of a much safer incision rather than the extensile lateral approach and long-term osseous stability that reduces the likelihood of developing further joint collapse, deformity, or Charcot neuroarthropathy. However, despite the advantages mentioned, this does not imply that all patients who are diabetic with peripheral neuropathy must undergo a primary subtalar joint fusion for management of intraarticular calcaneal fractures.

To perform a primary subtalar joint fusion via a limited sinus tarsi incision rather than an extensible lateral incision implies that the majority of the deformity to the calcaneus has been addressed. Often, these patients require a closed reduction under traction with percutaneous pinning to correct the calcaneal height, length, and frontal plane deformity to the tuberosity. Calcaneal width and a prominent lateral wall can easily be managed by performing a simple ostectomy through the same sinus tarsi incision that is used for a fusion and no further attempts of reduction other than manual compression need to be typically performed. For these reasons, the main focus of reduction is to correct frontal plane deformity while restoring the calcaneal height and length. Another alternative is to use external fixation, which is minimally invasive, to achieve traction and reduction. This temporary reduction is maintained for a minimum of 6 to 8 weeks at which time a primary subtalar joint fusion can be performed.

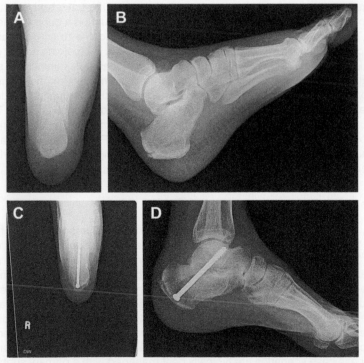

Fig. 3. Preoperative calcaneal axial (A) and lateral (B) radiographic views of closed calcaneal fracture in a patient with diabetes with dense peripheral neuropathy. Patient was casted and immobilized for 6 weeks before the primary subtalar joint fusion. Patient originally presented with venous stasis dermatitis, severe soft-tissue edema, and blisters. Final postoperative radiographs (C, D) showing primary subtalar joint fusion with a limited lateral approach and bone grafting at 7 months.

The surgical technique for performing an open reduction and primary subtalar joint fusion via an extensile lateral approach is identical to what was previously described with a few exceptions. The articular surface is removed from any fracture fragments of the calcaneus and from the posterior facet of the talus. In addition, the subchondral bone of the talus must be sufficiently drilled to induce vascular ingrowth across the fusion site. Fixation across the fusion site is typically achieved with one or two 6.5-mm cannulated screws that are either partially or fully threaded. Fully threaded screws are used when compression could lead to collapse. Often, autogenous or allogenic bone grafting is required for the calcaneal body and at the fusion site. Patients are kept non-weight bearing for a minimum of 10 to 12 weeks postoperatively to prevent malunion or nonunion.

MINIMAL APPROACH TO OPEN REDUCTION AND INTERNAL FIXATION

A minimal incisional approach to ORIF of calcaneal fractures is suitable for certain fracture patterns. Tongue type fractures that involve only two fracture fragments of the posterior facet can be attempted to be reduced using a minimal open incision. Essex-Lopresti[1] was the first to describe the technique to close reduce tongue type fractures of the calcaneus and used Steinman pins for fixation. Later, the technique was modified to incorporate placement of large cannulated screws or multiple small fragment screws that were placed percutaneously. On CT images the surgeon needs to determine if a large intraarticular fracture fragment is attached to the posterior superior calcaneal tuberosity confirming a tongue type fracture.

Patients are usually placed in a prone position on a radiolucent fracture table rather than a lateral decubitus position. The first step involves insertion of 3.2-mm guide pins just medial and lateral to the Achilles tendon into the posterior superior aspect of the calcaneal tuberosity and into the inferior aspect of the fracture fragment. The knee is then flexed to reduce the pull of the gastrocnemius soleus complex. After the fracture is mobilized, it can then be reduced and confirmed under fluoroscopic images on lateral, Broden, and calcaneal axial views. The second guide pin is advanced across the fracture into the plantar aspect of the anterior process. Once the fracture reduction is confirmed, 4.5- or 6.5-mm cannulated screws are placed over the guide pins. In some cases, additional 1.6-mm Steinmann pins will need to be inserted across the fracture line or the subtalar joint to maintain reduction.

At times, the fracture fragment may not reduce and a separate 2- to 3-cm incision needs to be made along the inferior aspect of the posterior facet of the subtalar joint. The incision is made about 1.5 cm inferior to the tip of the fibula, the peroneal sheath is incised and dissection is carried down to the lateral wall of the calcaneus between the peroneus brevis and longus tendons. Next, a curved elevator or small curved osteotome is used to gradually reflect the lateral wall and to identify the depressed articular surface. The fracture is then elevated and reduced and additional fixation can be provided with small fragment or cannulated screws from the lateral subchondral bone of the posterior facet into the sustentaculum tali. Bone graft can then be placed inferiorly to prevent later collapse and the lateral wall is tamped into the body of the calcaneus. Using this safe lateral incision is advantageous for initial fracture reduction, access for bone grafting, and to ensure that no gapping is present from the lateral to medial aspect and across the calcaneal articular surface.

EXTERNAL FIXATION FOR FRACTURE REDUCTION AND PRIMARY SUBTALAR JOINT FUSION

External fixation can also be used for primary calcaneal fracture reduction or subtalar joint arthrodesis. The use of a simple bar-to-clamp delta frame configuration or multiplane circular external fixation device are useful for management of selected calcaneal fractures.[12,13] The advantages of external fixation are numerous and some clinical case scenarios are discussed in detail later.

One clinical case scenario would involve an open and severely comminuted calcaneal fracture. Typically, a large wound is encountered along the posteromedial aspect of the calcaneus with severe fracture displacement of the medial wall. This would entail meticulous debridement and copious saline irrigation and closure if converted to a clean wound to prevent infection and to further facilitate later attempts at formal ORIF or conversion to a primary subtalar joint fusion, if possible. The use of external fixation allows the fracture fragments of the medial wall to be repositioned directly through the open wound while manipulating the calcaneal tuberosity with a half pin that may be later incorporated into the external fixation device maintaining the reduction to promote healing of the soft tissues. In addition, the external fixation device limits any joint motion that may induce tension on the compromised wound and surrounding soft tissues. The use of external fixation also allows easy access to evaluate the wound on a regular basis with little discomfort to patients. Pressure encountered from splints and casts may be detrimental for soft-tissue healing particularly when treating open fractures.

Furthermore, external fixation can be used for definitive management of either open or closed calcaneal fractures that are not amenable to open reduction and primary fusion with internal fixation. Typically these fractures display severe comminution with minimal cortical bone noted to the body of the calcaneus inferior to the subtalar joint. These calcaneal fractures present with the talus driven directly through the body of the calcaneus. For these cases, external fixation is advantageous to apply traction and fracture reduction through ligamentotaxis. For open fractures the joint can be approached directly through the open-fracture wound and prepared for arthrodesis. The posterior facet of the talar component of the subtalar joint is denuded of its cartilage and the subchondral plate is drilled to induced vascular ingrowth across the fusion site. Any visible soft-tissue interposition and remnants of articular surface are removed from the calcaneal bone defect. The large defect is bone grafted with either autogenous or allogenic corticocancellous bone. The bone graft that is inserted is allowed to consolidate and fuse to the talus while the external fixation device maintains the necessary reduction (**Fig. 4**). Closed fractures are managed with the same approach except a small 3-cm incision is required on the lateral aspect of the calcaneus and about 2 cm inferior to the tip of the fibula to access the subtalar joint for preparation of arthrodesis and for placement of the bone graft. Usually this requires the placement of an external fixation device for a minimum of 10 to 12 weeks.

Finally, external fixation use is ideal for calcaneal fracture management for patients who are not medically stable, are immunocompromised, or present with preexisting conditions that are relative or absolute contraindications for ORIF. These conditions can range from multi-trauma patients that present with multiple fractures to patients who are diabetic and neuropathic with multiple comorbidities. In these instances, the minimally invasive technique offered through a closed reduction under traction and application of an external fixation device is often a reasonable alternative. The authors tend to use this approach for patients in which simple casting and nonoperative fracture management will result in severe deformity that can potentially threaten patients' ability to resume an ambulatory status.

POSTOPERATIVE COMPLICATIONS AND MANAGEMENT

Calcaneal fracture management is associated with early and late complications.[14,15] Early complications of ORIF include wound dehiscence, necrosis, infection,

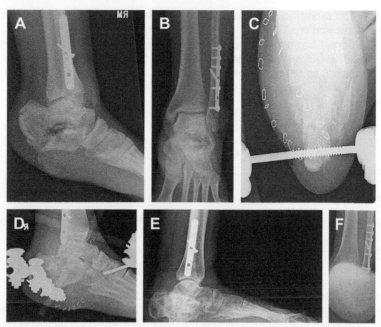

Fig. 4. Preoperative lateral foot (*A*) and ankle (*B*) radiographic views of an open calcaneal fracture with a severe degloving injury and comminution. Patient was brought immediately to the operating room for meticulous debridement and irrigation and stabilization with a delta external fixation configuration (*C, D*). Approximately 4 weeks after the operation the patient was brought back to the operating room for bone grafting of the calcaneal body and modification of the external fixation system. The fixation was removed at 10 weeks. Final postoperative radiographs (*E, F*) showing the outcome at 6 months.

neurovascular injury, thromboembolic events, and compartment syndrome. If a wound dehiscence is superficial, the surgeon may need to further immobilize the extremity and initiate local wound care and oral antibiotics. Full thickness skin necrosis or wound dehiscence with purulent drainage or underlying hematoma is better managed through surgical debridement, irrigation, parenteral antibiotics, and either local wound care or negative pressure wound therapy until definitive soft-tissue coverage is planned. Premature hardware removal and loss of fracture stabilization will further compromise the soft tissue, prevent infection control, and will most likely result in further complications. For these reasons and if osteomyelitis is suspected, it is paramount that a meticulous debridement is performed and the patients are placed on culture-specific intravenous antibiotics for at least 6 weeks based on intraoperative cultures and sensitivities. Hardware exposure usually requires a local flap or free tissue transfer. If the hardware is not exposed, negative pressure wound therapy is used until the wound heals secondarily or until a delayed primary closure can be performed.

Thromboembolic events and associated complications, although rare in foot and ankle surgery, are often underappreciated. The necessity of prophylaxis for deep vein thrombosis (DVT) in patients who undergo foot and ankle surgery remains undefined. The compound effect of surgery, trauma, and prolonged immobilization place these patients at risk for DVT and, although rare, pulmonary embolism.

Compartment syndrome in association with calcaneal fractures has also been documented. Most reported cases involved the subcalcaneal compartment. Early recognition and prompt decompression of the affected compartment is essential to avoid late complications.

Further reported complications associated with surgical management of calcaneal fractures include, but are not limited to, hardware failure, malunion, nonunion, post-traumatic arthritis, and nerve injury.[14–16]

SUMMARY

Appropriate procedure selection and prompt timing of surgery are important factors in obtaining a successful outcome. Use of these current approaches to the surgical management of calcaneal fractures is essential to minimize early and late complications.

REFERENCES

1. Essex-Lopresti P. The mechanism, reduction technique, and results in fractures of the os calcis. Br J Surg 1952;39:395–419.
2. Sanders R, Fortin P, DiPasquale A, et al. Operative treatment in 120 displaced intra-articular fractures of the calcaneus. Results using a prognostic computed tomographic scan classification. Clin Orthop 1993;290:87–95.
3. Buckley R, Tough S, McCormack R, et al. Operative compared with nonoperative treatment of displaced intra-articular calcaneal fractures:a prospective, randomized, controlled multicenter trial. J Bone Joint Surg Am 2002;84:1733–44.
4. Benirschke SK, Sangeorzan BJ, Hansen ST. Extensive intraarticular fractures of the foot. Surgical management of calcaneal fractures. Clin Orthop 1993;292:128–34.
5. Bezes H, Massart P, Delvaux D, et al. The operative treatment of intraarticular calcaneal fractures, Indications, technique, and results in 257 cases. Clin Orthop 1993;290:55–9.
6. Cotton F, Henderson F. Results of fractures of the os calcis. Am J Orthop Surg 1916;14:290.
7. Zwipp H. Reconstructive surgery of malunited joint fractures of the foot. Orthopade 1990;19(6):409–15.
8. Myerson M, Quill GE Jr. Late complications of fractures of the calcaneus. J Bone Joint Surg Am 1993;75(3):331–41.
9. Romash MM. Calcaneal fractures: three-dimensional treatment. Foot Ankle 1988; 8(4):180–97.
10. Buckley RE, Tough S. Displaced intra-articular calcaneal fractures. J Am Acad Orthop Surg 2004;12(3):172–8.
11. Buch BD, Myerson MS, Miller SD. Primary subtalar arthrodesis for the treatment of comminuted calcaneal fractures. Foot Ankle Int 1996;17:61–70.
12. Zgonis T, Roukis TS, Polyzois VD. The use of Ilizarov technique and other types of external fixation for the treatment of intra-articular calcaneal fractures. Clin Podiatr Med Surg 2006;23:343–53.
13. Roukis TS, Wunschel M, Lutz HP, et al. Treatment of displaced intra-articular calcaneal fracture with triangular tube-to-bar external fixation: long term clinical follow-up and radiographic analysis. Clin Podiatr Med Surg 2008;28:285–99.
14. Sangeorzan BJ. Salvage procedures for calcaneus fractures. Instr Course Lect 1997;46:339–46.
15. Walter JH Jr, Rockett MS, Goss LR. Complications of intra-articular fractures of the calcaneus. J Am Podiatr Med Assoc 2004;94(4):382–8.
16. Stapleton JJ, Belczyk R, Zgonis T. Surgical treatment of calcaneal fracture malunions and posttraumatic deformities. Clin Podiatr Med Surg 2009;26:79–90.

Complications of Heel Surgery

George F. Wallace, DPM, MBA

KEYWORDS

• Complications • Heel surgery • Calcaneus • Foot and ankle

Complication is defined as "A morbid process or event occurring during a disease that is not an essential part of the disease, although it may result from it or from independent causes."[1] Using this definition, foot and ankle surgeons would substitute the words, *surgery* or *surgical procedure*, for the word, *disease*. Anyone who relates having no complications can be accused of not doing surgery, not recognizing them, or failing to acknowledge their occurrence. There are myriad surgical procedures performed on the calcaneus for a variety of pathologies (**Table 1**). Everyone has a potential for a complication no matter how well surgery is performed. In a broad sense, complications can be characterized as being iatrogenic or resulting from a breach in patient compliance. The latter can be avoided to an extent with perioperative education and frequent reminders about following directions.

Any of the complications (discussed later) have to be discovered early. They need to be addressed promptly. Candid discussion with patients regarding complications and what is required to fix a problem is necessary. Keeping patients ill informed or misinformed or burying one's head in the sand is inappropriate. How foot and ankle surgeons apply the rule to be open and acknowledge a complication may make the difference between a medical malpractice suit initiated or an incident falling just under the complication rubric.

SURGICAL PLANNING

No matter how meticulously a surgical intervention is planned, statistically a complication can ensue. As Louis Pasteur famously said, "Chance favors the prepared mind."[2] Proper preparation can lessen the chance of a complication. All the planning in the world, however, can never eliminate a complication.

Planning begins with an accurate history and physical examination. Comorbidities, such as diabetes, osteoporosis, and rheumatoid arthritis, have to be taken

Podiatry Service, University Hospital – University of Medicine and Dentistry of New Jersey, 150 Bergen Street, G-142, Newark, NJ 07103, USA
E-mail address: wallacgf@umdnj.edu

Clin Podiatr Med Surg 27 (2010) 393–406
doi:10.1016/j.cpm.2010.04.001

Table 1
Common surgical procedures performed on the calcaneus
Resection of exostoses from various locations
Haglund deformity resection
Calcaneal osteotomies
ORIF of calcaneal fractures
Arthrodeses
Tumor resection
Miscellaneous

into account. These may not lead directly to complications but can increase their rate. Vigilance within the postoperative period then becomes paramount. Smoking history has to be factored in also. If surgery is required after a traumatic episode, or a "redo" surgery is performed, foot and ankle surgeons must know how these can affect complications. The diagnosis of the pathology has to be accurate. Surgical procedures matches the pathology and the patients' medical condition and psyche. Surgeon experience for the index procedures should be within a comfortable framework. Experience in something as complex as open reduction internal fixation (ORIF) of a calcaneal fracture improves outcomes due to the steep learning curve.[3]

Templates may be used to facilitate surgical performance. Saw bones can be used for practice. Reconstructions in 3-D allow for a better understanding of fracture patterns and spatial relationships (**Fig. 1**).

All these steps are repeated when faced with a complication requiring additional surgery. Surgical intervention to fix a complication, however, can create patient and surgeon angst. The surgeon is cognizant of the previously operated soft tissue envelope, scar tissue, bone composition, fixation, and systemic factors that have an impact on eliminating the complication. Rarely can the foot withstand multiple attempts before a patient is classified a "surgical foot cripple."[4] Each surgery adds extended healing times to recuperation.

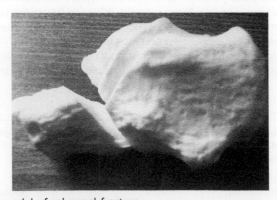

Fig. 1. Saw bone model of calcaneal fracture.

TAXONOMY OF COMPLICATIONS

For the purpose of this discussion, a taxonomy system is proposed. This system groups complications as follows

1. Cause
   - Iatrogenic
   - Compliance issues
2. Temporal
   - Immediate
   - Late
3. Location
   - Contiguous
   - Distal to surgical site.

Compliance issues result purely from a patient's own behavior, whether or not willful. A patient's compliance can range from falling on the surgical extremity, which disrupts the internal fixation, to not remaining non–weight bearing in spite of instructions to do so. Unfortunately, the degree of compliance cannot be measured preoperatively. Although iatrogenic connotes (incorrectly) pure physician input, more precisely, it is a response to the surgery, induced by the surgery itself. Iatrogenic can be construed as within any segment of medical care.[5] Iatrogenic results are not automatically considered malpractice.

Immediate complications occur within a short time period. Three weeks is used in this article. Examples are a postoperative infection, loss of fixation, and deep vein thrombosis (DVT). Late complications are those occurring more than 3 weeks from the surgical date. Examples are a nonunion or malunion. There can be overlap as in loss of fixation.

Contiguous complications manifest directly at the surgical site. Infection and dehiscence are examples. Distal complications (ie, far removed from the surgical site) diagnoses are DVT or cast disease.

INFECTION

For this discussion, the surgical procedures on the calcaneus are clean cases. The rate of infection for clean cases in foot and ankle surgery has been reported as 2.2%.[6] ORIF of calcaneal fractures, however, can lead to a higher infection rate.[7] Concomitant medical diagnoses also can affect the infection rate.

There are 2 basic types of infection: superficial and deep. The former may present as cellulitis or as a superficial abscess, managed, for the most part, on an outpatient basis. The extent of the cellulitis, lymphangitis/adinopathy, or systemic signs dictate whether or not a superficial infection is more serious. A deep infection requires hospitalization, intravenous antibiotics, and formal incision and drainage. The goal of any infection is to prevent direct extension osteomyelitis.[8]

Arbeitsgemeinschaft für Osteosynthesefragen (German for *Association for the Study of Internal Fixation*) (AO) principles dictate retaining internal fixation in the presence of an infection if stability of the osseous construct and fixation is maintained (**Fig. 2**).[9] If not, then loose screws and plates are removed and fixation is usually changed to an external fixation device while the bone heals. Pins for these are placed well away from any infection so as to not seed bacteria when drilling.

The advent of methicillin-resistant *Staphlococcus aureus* (MRSA) infections, hospital and community acquired, are rapidly increasing in presentation.[10] A high

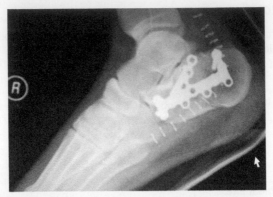

Fig. 2. Hardware retained in presence of infection if stable; not loose.

index of suspicion that MRSA organisms are present is paramount when an infection occurs. Antibiotics are selected with this in mind.

Immune status and comorbidities gleaned from the history could play a role not only in the appearance of an infection but also in how it is treated. An example is a diabetic who may not present with a leukocytosis or general malaise.

Proper surgical principles can go a long way to improving outcome. Meticulous tissue handling, absence of dead space, expeditious surgical times, timing and judicious use of perioperative antibiotics, and experience lower the probability of an infection.[11]

External fixator components, which penetrate the skin, inserted initially or later on because of a complication, can also be the source of infection. Pin tract infections are common. Loose and improperly inserted pins are etiologic factors. Pin tracts are examined during each visit. The area is cleaned. Daily pin tract care does not prove more beneficial than weekly care.[12] The prevention of direct extension osteomyelitis and of pin loosening are the goals of keeping pin tracts infection-free.

LOSS OF FIXATION

Calcaneal surgery in many instances requires some type of fixation. Proper fixation techniques begin when the osteotomy or arthrodesis is created. Bone stock can dictate fixation type. Osteopenic bone may not hold screws. Diabetics, especially if neuropathic, should have additional points of fixation.

The advent of intraoperative fluoroscopy creates a real-time status of fixation. Immediate postoperative flat plate radiographs, however, should continue to be obtained. Any deviation may necessitate a return to the operating room on an emergent basis (**Fig. 3**). Serial radiographs are taken whenever there is a change in weight-bearing status to monitor osseous healing or if there are clinical suspicions that an untoward effect has occurred.[13]

Patient compliance plays a large role in determining that the intended outcome is achieved. Patients need to be fully informed of the surgery, perioperative requirements, and the length of time required to resume shoe wear and activities. For use with external fixation, the author has coined a simple but profound phrase, "The size of the frame must match the frame of the mind."

Loss of fixation entails a prompt response when discovered. Treatment options include new fixation systems, repositioning if bone migration, prolonged

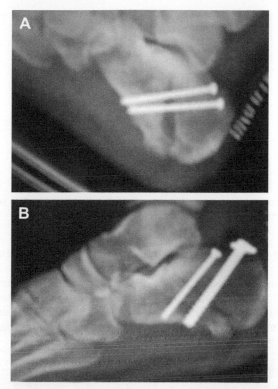

Fig. 3. (*A*) Calcaneal fracture fixated. Patient while in the recovery room put weight on foot causing displacement. (*B*) Immediately returned to surgery with new fixation.

immobilization, and non–weight bearing. As discussed previously, loss of fixation can be a result of an infection.

Painful hardware or screws that are backing out are removed. The construct has to be healed, however, before extirpation. Protected weight bearing follows removal due to the stress risers created with fixation detachment.[14] Of concern are the screws placed in the posteroplantar calcaneus for an osteotomy or subtalar fusion. Although this may be a better construct, if not placed correctly, the screw heads can cause pain when weight bearing or from shoe irritation (**Fig. 4**).

OVERCORRECTION AND UNDERCORRECTION

Calcaneal surgery, for the most part, does not deal with simply removing a subcutaneous soft tissue mass in toto then calling it a day. Instead, due to the pathology of the calcaneus itself or the correction of a deformity, heel surgery requires some kind of correction first and fixation/arthrodesis second. Although patients and surgeons aim for the best results, there is always the possibility of undercorrection (ie, not resecting enough of a retrocalcaneal exostosis) or overcorrection (ie, a subtalar fusion in many degrees of valgus).

Surgeons have to plan surgery in a meticulous way. Templates may be used as guides. The diagnosis is only formalized when all diagnostic modalities are exhausted. For example, a CT scan is ordered when a calcaneal fracture is diagnosed (**Fig. 5**).

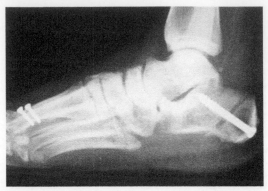

Fig. 4. Screw placed to secure a medial calcaneal slide osteotomy. The screw head is irritating in surgical boot and shoes.

Plain films include a calcaneal axial in addition to the three standard views. Following is an illustration.

A 52-year-old Hispanic woman was initially seen with heel pain. Plantar fasciitis with plantar calcaneal exostosis was the diagnosis. Conservative management was initiated. The patient returned to her country for resection of the exostosis. After a prolonged recovery, she returned and presented with continued heel pain. Radiographs

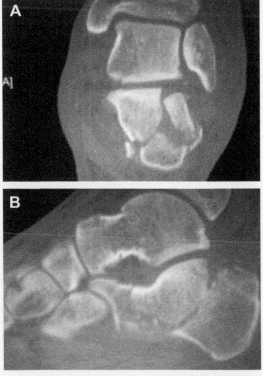

Fig. 5. CT scans of calcaneal fracture. (A) Coronal view. (B) Sagittal view.

revealed a calcaneal fracture along with an overly aggressive heel spur resection (**Fig. 6**). At this time, she refused further surgery. Subsequently, she was sent to the orthotist for evaluation and fabrication of a patellar weight-bearing device.

Even though overcorrection or undercorrection may be apparent on radiographs, patients can be asymptomatic and function adequately. In such a case, the radiograph is not treated nor can they ever be. The films, along with any subjective complaints, are a different story and must be addressed appropriately. **Table 2** lists some of the over- and undercorrection scenarios that can be encountered. Being adept with the surgical procedure from experience can facilitate more favorable outcomes.[3]

NONUNION

Due to the high cancellous bone content within the calcaneus, the rate of nonunions is low when looking at osteotomies. Nonunions can occur, however, especially when performing an arthrodesis. Subtalar arthrodeses have various nonunion rates reported.[15,16] Although rare, nonunions can occur with calcaneal fractures.[17]

Nonunions are caused by many factors. Some of them are noncompliance, failure of fixation, smoking, poor bone quality, diabetes, infection, steroid use, and various immunocompromised conditions.[18] Two definitions are used for nonunions. Insurance issues may dictate which one is used. The more traditional definition of a nonunion is when there is no bone healing at 6 to 8 months.[19] A more practical definition of a nonunion is when there is no evidence of any osseous healing for 3 consecutive months.[20] The latter can shorten the time for rendering a diagnosis of nonunion. Nonunions are classified as hypertrophic or atrophic. Each is then subdivided. The shape of the calcaneus does not lend itself to easily characterizing the type of nonunion.

Besides plain films, a triphasic technetium Tc 99m bone scan is obtained. Three patterns are distinctive: uptake across the operative osseous site signifying a hypertrophic nonunion, no uptake on either side representing an atrophic nonunion, and uptake again on both sides with cold cleft in the middle. The last example represents a pseudoarthrosis.

Hypertrophic nonunions may simply need better or prolonged immobilization. Atrophic nonunions require surgical intervention. The osseous interfaces are débrided to raw bleeding bone (paprika sign). A bone graft may be inserted when the gap is too large for simple opposition.

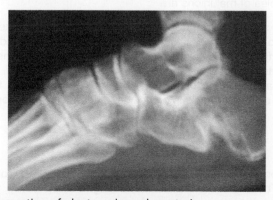

Fig. 6. Aggressive resection of plantar calcaneal exostosis.

Table 2
Over- and undercorrection of common surgical precedures performed on the calcaneus

Procedure	Overcorrection	Undercorrection
Plantar heel spur resection	Gouging; fracture plantar cortex	Minimal to no bone removed[a]
Retrocalcaneal exostectomy; Haglund deformity	Grouping; extensive loss of calcaneal architecture	Residual bone, especially impeding tendon function
ORIF valcaneal fractures	Excessive valgus of tuberosity fragment	Lateral wall blow out not reduced; varus of tuberosity fragment; poor fixation; facets with step off[a]
Arthrodesis	Creation of new deformity in "opposite direction"	Deformity not completely corrected
Calcaneal osteotomies	Creation of new deformity in "opposite direction"	Deformity not completely corrected

[a] Not necessary to remove bone at all.

Nonunions can be prevented somewhat by fostering patient compliance, smoking cessation, adequate fixation, and good surgical principles. Due to the complex nature of most calcaneal surgeries, there are enhancements that can be used. These fall in the categories of orthobiologics and bone stimulators. Nothing can replace using autografts when that option is possible. Orthobiologic devices are expensive and may encounter insurance resistance. Applying bone stimulators immediately after surgery in a prophylactic mode may also not meet insurance approval. The surgeon may have to wait until a delayed union is diagnosed for use.

In some instances, a nonunion may be present on plain films; however, patients experience no pain at all. Patients must be properly informed. Further treatment may hinge on a complaint of discomfort in the area.

MALUNION

A malunion can be encountered whenever the osteotomy or fusion site heals in a position that is not intended. This can result in under- or overcorrection. Unless symptomatic, malunions can be observed. Should symptoms arise, then the malunion is corrected. Examples of malunions are

1. The proverbial subtalar arthrodesis fused in varus. This most likely causes lateral column symptoms and possibly chronic ankle sprains. Similar findings could occur where internal fixation of a calcaneal fracture is attempted and the tuberosity fragment is not reduced out of varus.
2. A medial calcaneal sliding osteotomy, whereby the posterior fragment subsequently tilts or shifts and heals in a position not conducive to proper weight distribution (**Fig. 7**).

DVT

The immobilization routinely used after calcaneal surgery is a factor in the development of DVT. The incidence varies depending on the study and procedures analyzed.[21,22]

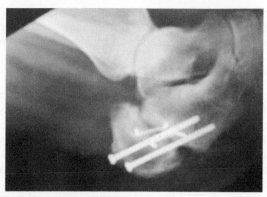

Fig. 7. Early weight bearing after a medial calcaneal slide osteotomy. Loss of fixation and shifting of osteotomy.

Some have advocated that a calf thrombus does not have to be treated because of the low incidence of propagation into a pulmonary embolus.[23,24] A question arises: If a calf thrombus does propagate, the first stop is in the more proximal leg veins, which then has a far greater chance of dislodging and creating a pulmonary embolus—should this be a reason to treat? At the University of Medicine and Dentistry of New Jersey (UMDNJ)–University Hospital a calf thrombus is aggressively treated.

Through patients' medical history, a predilection can be determined for a DVT. The surgery itself, a previous diagnosis of DVT, malignancy, oral contraceptives, blood dyscrasias, and obesity are factors.[25] With any of these, prophylaxis is instituted. Intraoperatively, this may preclude the use of any tourniquet. On the contralateral extremity, antithrombolic devices are put on. Postoperatively, antithrombotic stockings on the contralateral limb are kept in place and ankle exercises and subcutaneous enoxaparin sodium are administered. Patients may even be discharged with a prescription for enoxaparin sodium and instructions on how to administer it. Patients requiring overnight stays are routinely administered enoxaparin sodium as prophylaxis for DVT.

Whenever patients are examined postoperatively, in the office or during hospital rounds, they are asked whether or not they are experiencing any calf tenderness. Also, the calves are squeezed to elicit tenderness. Should any of the aforementioned steps prove positive, calf circumference can then be measured. Or, as is the case at University Hospital–UMDNJ, the patients are sent for noninvasive duplex venous scans. This is a quick way to determine if there is a thrombosis. Wolf and colleagues[26] hold anticoagulation if negative. Equivocal findings can always be adjudicated using the diagnostic gold standard, venography. Although D-dimer evaluations can be measured, they are not routinely used at UMDNJ–University Hospital. If measured, a negative D-dimer test rules out the diagnosis of DVT.[27,28]

The index of suspicion for a DVT when presented with calf tenderness should be high. Waiting for redness, palpable chords, or increase in calf circumference delays diagnosis and ultimately treatment. An analogy can be used to illustrate. A patient with chest pain presenting to an emergency department has a routine EKG performed. Many times the cause is noncardiac and the EKG is negative. Calf findings, akin to the chest pain, undergo a noninvasive duplex venous scan to rule in or out the DVT, which is a simplistic approach to a complex entity.

Ultimately, preventing a pulmonary embolus is the goal. Postoperative patients with a pulmonary embolus may never exhibit any thrombotic symptoms or findings.

Postoperative shortness of breath, diaphoresis, and general malaise in the absence of primarily an infection alerts physicians to a pulmonary embolism until proved otherwise. In some instances, death may be the sole finding of the pulmonary embolism.[29]

COMPLEX REGIONAL PAIN SYNDROME

Complex regional pain syndrome (CRPS) does not have a predilection for calcaneal surgery but it must be included in any discussion. Although surgery can lead to this chronic pain syndrome, any kind of trauma, even minor, can develop into CRPS.[30]

Decades ago, CRPS was lumped under the rubric of reflex sympathetic dystrophy. In 1995, the current classification of CRPS was formulated.[31] CRPS I is the old reflex sympathetic dystrophy, wherein a named nerve is not directly traumatized. CRPS II, or causalgia, is from a direct injury to a specific nerve.

An index of suspicion is needed for postoperative calcaneal surgical patients who present with unremitting pain, pain out of proportion to the surgery, prolonged pain, and physical changes characteristic of CRPS (**Table 3**).[32] In a personal communication with a pain specialist, he found throughout his career that, as a whole, podiatric surgeons referred patients to determine the presence of CRPS at a later time than their orthopaedics counterparts (Andrew Kaufman, MD, personal communication, 2009). This is somewhat perplexing when an earlier diagnosis can yield a more rapid and successful outcome.[33] Therefore, it is prudent to obtain a pain consultation to rule in or out CRPS at the earliest time.

Various treatments have proved beneficial in combating CRPS.[34] Besides a prompt diagnosis, mobilization has been shown important in treatment. The psychological component should not be overlooked.[35]

How can CRPS be explained to patients? Technical jargon may confuse or tune out individuals with CRPS. The following analogy is based on one of the theories of CRPS formation, the gate control theory of pain, by Melzak and Wael[36]:

> Pain is started by a traumatic event, in this case, surgery. The pain gate is open. Analgesics, physical therapy, and the body itself close the gate and then pain subsides. For reasons not known, in some individuals, the pain gate stays partially or completely open, hence, the diagnosis of CRPS. Everything used from this point on is an attempt to close the gate.

Periodically, patients may be encountered who present with a history of CRPS and need calcaneal surgery. Anesthesia is notified regarding these patients. Such patients

Table 3 CRPS
Types
I—Reflex sympathetic dystrophy
II—Causalgia
Clinical Findings
Neuropathic pain
Edema
Trophic skin changes
Loss of joint motion
Vasomotor changes
Radiographic signs

are more susceptible to a repeat CRPS episode. These cases require an epidural anesthesia for pain control, gentle mobilization, and patient-controlled analgesics. A popliteal block could also be administered.

How about patients who do not have CRPS but continue to have chronic pain after exhausting all diagnostic and treatment options? Unfortunately, these patients have little recourse but to manage any remnants of pain after the surgery as best as possible. Whatever pain, edema, or other untoward symptoms linger after 1 year, patients must understand that this situation most likely is permanent.

CHARCOT ARTHROPATHY

It is not uncommon, with the explosion in numbers of diabetic patients, to perform surgery for a calcaneal fracture or something more elective. The iatrogenic trauma of surgery or community-acquired trauma, especially in neuropathic patients, can predispose to developing an acute Charcot arthropathy presentation.

Included in any physical examination for diabetes is the establishment of the presence of normal sensation. Any decrease is noted along with subjective statements of numbness or paresthesias. When encountered, surgeons plan accordingly. This may take the form of extrafixation and doubling the time required for fracture/osteotomy healing.[37] In those non–weight-bearing patients, the contralateral limb is always assessed and protected for Charcot arthropathy development. Additionally, casts are changed frequently not only for wound inspection but also to inhibit irritation and subsequent ulceration on bony prominences from cast slippage or snugness.

A red, hot edematous foot with pain somewhat out of proportion to degree of neuropathy diagnosed alerts to the possibility of an acute Charcot arthropathy. Other considerations in the differential are infection and an acute gout attack if the latter is within the history.

Once a diagnosis of Charcot arthropathy is made, appropriate treatments are initiated. The mainstay is immobilization and non–weight bearing. Bisphosphanate therapy may be part of the treatment protocol.[38]

CAST DISEASE

Cast disease encompasses the triad of calf atrophy, joint stiffness, and osteopenia.[39] Calcaneal surgery usually requires a prolonged time in a cast or rigid immobilizer. Patients are made aware of the adverse consequences but reassured that measures will be undertaken to establish normal muscle mass, full range of motion, and reverse osteopenia.

The mainstay of therapy for cast disease is physical therapy. The sooner physical therapy begins, the quicker cast disease is erased. Whether or not patients understand the goals of physical therapy, they must be motivated and compliant to accomplish the goals established before the initiation of the therapy.

A frank discussion regarding the diagnosis, surgical procedures, and postoperative course is necessary before surgical intervention. Although it cannot be predicted with accuracy how long it will take before return to full activity and wearing shoes, there should be, nonetheless, a reasonable estimation. For example, a surgeon would never say after ORIF of a calcaneal fracture that a patient will be healed and back in shoes in 3 weeks. This is unreasonable and paints too rosy a picture. A more realistic time frame, 8 to 10 weeks, conveys a more sensible approach. Foot and ankle surgeons should give periodic updates of when the time goals will be met.

LEGAL ISSUES

A complication of any surgery in general, and on the calcaneus specifically, is not considered malpractice. Unfortunately, complications or bad results do occur. These are far different from those situations when gross negligence has occurred; for example, when the posterior tibial tendon is transected performing a calcaneal osteotomy, it is not recognized intraoperatively and never diagnosed postoperatively or ignored in spite of patient complaints and muscular imbalances.

In rapid sequence, a complication can turn into a legal predicament if a patient assumes something is being hidden, a rosy picture is presented in spite of evidence to the contrary, nothing is explained, or there is a nagging insistence regarding payment. Therefore, nothing should be hidden or downplayed, and blame should not be shifted to a patient. Foot and ankle surgeons must explain in detail the complication, render a plausible explanation one has occurred, and offer a way to remedy the situation.

When faced with a complication, a second opinion should never be discouraged if mentioned. Sometimes, a surgeon may initiate the seeking of another opinion.

The following are important steps from a medical/legal perspective[40,41]:

1. The consent is accurate, spelling out the procedure and complications. Hospitals and surgicenters each have an institutional consent. If one feels a consent is inadequate then a more detailed consent can be composed through the surgeon's office. This is in addition to the institution's.
2. Conservative options have been tried and exhausted. A patient's chart reflects this.
3. The surgery is appropriate for the pathology and is within the standard of care.
4. The surgery is within the scope of privileges granted by the institution and, equally important, within the foot and ankle surgeon's scope of training.
5. If served a summons, be professional and cooperative at all times.
6. NEVER alter a chart!
7. Notify the insurance carrier as soon as possible if a suit is served.
8. Cooperate with the legal team assigned by the insurance carrier.

The reflex action with any complication is to sweep it under the rug hoping it goes away. Luckily, experience and training take over so the complication can be dealt with in an expeditious manner.

A special predicament is rendering a second opinion in light of a colleague's less than optimal result. This is a difficult situation. Bhattacharyya and Yeon[42] provide cogent guidelines for dealing with this. In some instances, the second foot and ankle surgeon takes on the additional burden of performing corrective surgery.

NEWER DEVELOPMENTS

There are some developments that may play an ever-increasing role in the analysis of postoperative complications.

Fayad and colleagues[43] looked at the use of 3-D CT in evaluating complications of hardware. They were able to show examples of this modality versus plain films and conventional CT. If 3-D CT is available, it should be used for infection, fractured/painful hardware, malplacement, and loosening.

Richter and Zech[44] investigated the use of intraoperative pedobarography to modify positions of various arthrodeses. Although their numbers were small, there were improved outcome scores when compared with a cohort not using the device where the position of arthrodesis was never altered from a biomechanical function. Possibly, the pedobarograph may be a fixture in surgical theaters and routinely used.

SUMMARY

Surgical complications of the calcaneus are unique to that structure but do not have a greater incidence than in any other part of the foot or ankle. The first tenet of any complication, however, is to recognize it. When all is said and done, recognition is probably the most important step when a complication arises.

REFERENCES

1. Spraycar M, editor. Stedman's medical dictionary. 26 edition. Baltimore (MD): Williams & Wilkins; 1995. p. 375.
2. Selders G, editor. The great thoughts. New York: Ballantine Books; 1985. p. 324.
3. Johnson RW, Benirschke SK, Carr JB, et al. Symposium: the treatment of displaced intraarticular fractures of the calcaneus. Contemp Orthop 1996;32(3): 187–207.
4. Johnson KA. The surgical foot cripple and quackery. In: Surgery of the foot and ankle. New York: Raven Press; 1989. p. 281–94.
5. Leiyu S, Singh DA. Outpatient and primary care services. In: Leiyu S, Singh DA, Shi I, editors. Delivering health care in America. A systems approach. 3rd edition. Sudbury (MA): Jones and Bartlett; 2004.
6. Miller WA. Postoperative wound infection in foot and ankle surgery. Foot Ankle 1983;4:102–4.
7. Court-Brown CM, Schmidt M, Schutte BG. Factors affecting infection after calcaneal fracture fixation. Injury 2009;40(12):1313–5.
8. Lazz Arini L, Mader JT, Calhoun JH. Osteomyelitis in long bones. J Bone Joint Surg Am 2004;86(10):2305–18.
9. Ochsner PE, Sirkin MS, Trampuz A. Acute infection. In: Ruedi TP, Buckley RE, Moran CG, editors. AO principles of fracture management. 2nd edition. New York: Thieme; 2007. p. 521–40.
10. Patel A, Calfee RP, Plante M, et al. Methicillin-resistant staphylococcus aureus in orthopaedic surgery. J Bone Joint Surg Br 2008;90(11):1401–6.
11. Stapp MD, Taylor RP. Edema, hematoma, and infection. In: Banks AS, Downey MS, Martin DE, et al, editors. McGlamry's comprehensive textbook of foot and ankle surgery. 3rd edition. Philadelphia: Lippincott Williams Wilkins; 2001. p. 1997–2015.
12. Parameswaran AD, Roberts CS, Seligson D, et al. Pin tract infection with contemporary external fixation: how much of a problem? J Orthop Trauma 2003;17(7): 503–7.
13. Gerbert J, Albin RL, Borrelli A, et al. Adult dysfunctional flatfoot. American College of Foot and Ankle Surgeons preferred practice guideline. 1997. p. 1–34.
14. Alford JW, Bradley MP, Fadale PD, et al. Resorbable fillers reduce stress risers from empty screw holes. J Trauma 2007;63(3):647–54.
15. Child BJ, Hix J, Catanzariti AR, et al. The effect of hindfoot realignment in triple arthrodesis. J Foot Ankle Surg 2009;48(3):285–93.
16. Chahal J, Stephen DJ, Bilmer B, et al. Factors associated with outcome after subtalar arthrodesis. J Orthop Trauma 2006;20(8):555–61.
17. Schepers T, Batka P. Calcaneal nonunions: three cases and a review of the literature. Arch Orthop Trauma Surg 2008;128(7):735–8.
18. Asseous M, Bhamra MS. Should os calcis fractures in smokers be fixed? A review of 40 patients. Injury 2001;32(8):631–2.
19. Panagiotis M. Classification of nonunion. Injury 2005;36(Suppl 4):30–7.

20. Hernigou P, Poignard A, Beaujean F, et al. Percutaneous autologus bone-marrow grafting for non-union. J Bone Joint Surg Am 2005;87(7):1430–7.
21. Wells PS, Owen C, Doucette S, et al. Does this patient have deep vein thrombosis? JAMA 2006;295(2):199–207.
22. Solis G, Saxby T. Incidence of DVT following surgery of the foot and ankle. Foot Ankle Int 2002;23(5):411–4.
23. Righini M, Bounameaux H. Clinical relevance of distal vein thrombosis. Curr Opin Pulm Med 2008;14(5):408–13.
24. Cohen AT, Balaratnam S, Fassaladis N. Are isolated distal deep vein thromboses clinically significant? Therapy 2008;5(2):151–7.
25. Galanaud JP, Quenet S, Rivron-Guillot K, et al. Comparison of the clinical history of symptomatic isolated distal deep-vein thrombosis in 11086 patients (RIERE registry). J Thromb Haemost 2009;7(12):2028–34.
26. Wolf B, Nicholas DM, Duncan JL. Safety of a single duplex scan to exclude deep vein thrombosis. Br J Surg 2000;87(11):1525–8.
27. Jenersjo CM, Fagerberg IH, Karlander SG, et al. Normal d-dimer concentration is a common finding in symptomatic outpatients with distal deep vein thrombosis. Blood Coagul Fibrinolysis 2005;16(7):517–23.
28. Kelly J, Rudd A, Lewis RR. Plasma d-dimer in the diagnosis of venous thrombo-embolism. Arch Intern Med 2002;162(7):747–56.
29. Hirsh J, Bates SM. Prognosis in acute pulmonary embolism. Lancet 1999; 353(9162):1375–6.
30. Harris J, Fallat L, Schwartz S. Characteristic trends of lower extremity complex regional pain syndrome. J Foot Ankle Surg 2004;43(5):296–301.
31. Stanton-Hicks M, Janig W, Hassenbusch S, et al. Reflex sympathetic dystrophy: changing concepts and taxonomy. Pain 1995;63(1):127–33.
32. Atkins RM. Aspects of current management. Complex regional pain syndrome. J Bone Joint Surg Br 2003;85(8):1100–6.
33. Reuben SS. Preventing the development of complex regional pain syndrome after surgery. Anesthesiology 2004;101(5):1215–24.
34. Kingery WS. A critical review of controlled clinical trials for peripheral neuropathic pain and complex regional pain syndrome. Pain 1997;73(2):123–39.
35. Weisberg JN, Vaillancourt PD. Personality factors and disorders in chronic pain. Semin Clin Neuropsychiatry 1999;4(3):155–66.
36. DeLeo JA. Basic science of pain. J Bone Joint Surg Am 2006;88(2):558–62.
37. Holmes GB Jr, Hill N. Fractures and dislocations of the foot and ankle in diabetes associated with Charcot joint changes. Foot Ankle Int 1994;15(4):182–5.
38. Jude EB. Pharmacological management of the acute Charcot foot. Foot Ankle Q Sem J 2007;19(2):51–7.
39. Halanski M, Noonan KJ. Cast and splint immobilization: complications. J Am Acad Orthop Surg 2008;16(1):30–40.
40. Bunch W. Informed consent. Clin Orthop Relat Res 2000;378(1):71–7.
41. Easley ME. Medicolegal aspects of foot and ankle surgery. Clin Orthop Relat Res 2005;433(9):77–81.
42. Bhattacharyya T, Yeon H. Doctor, was this surgery done wrong? J Bone Joint Surg Am 2005;87(1):223–5.
43. Fayad LM, Patra A, Fishman EK. Value of 3D CT in defining skeletal complications of orthopedic hardware in the postoperative patient. AJR Am J Roentgenol 2009; 193(10):1155–63.
44. Richter M, Zech S. Intraoperative pedobarography leads to improved outcome scores: a level 1 study. Foot Ankle Int 2009;30(11):1029–36.

Dermatologic Causes of Heel Pain

George F. Wallace, DPM, MBA

KEYWORDS

• Dermatology • Plantar verrucae • Intractable plantar keratosis
• Heel fissures

Although many patients with heel pain have a diagnosis that is not related to the skin, there are entities that the foot and ankle surgeon has to be aware of and include in the differential diagnosis. Some entities may be subtle, such as an intractable plantar keratosis (IPK), whereas others, such as heel fissures, may be readily visible. The dermatologic causes of heel pain should not be trivialized.

Some of the dermatologic diagnoses may eventually lead to surgery if conservative measures fail. Plantar verruca is included in this category. Others, such as an IPK, may have an underlying bony exostosis as the causative agent, which would need to be resected for resolution of the keratosis.

This article describes some of the more common pathologies. They are not presented in order of prevalence or severity.

As with any patient's subjective complaint, a thorough history and physical examination is fundamental to a diagnosis. The physician most likely will use the familiar NLDOCAT pneumonic. The dermatologic aspects of this are:

N : Nature

Size, appearance, stages, symptomatology associated with the lesion

L : Location

On a weight-bearing surface; on the contralateral foot in a mirror image location, on another part(s) of the body

D : Duration

How long has the lesion been present? Are there new ones that have recently appeared?

O : Onset

What, if anything, precipitated the lesion to occur, or what aggravates it at this time?

C : Course

How has the lesion progressed; has it evolved or enlarged?

Podiatry Service, University Hospital – University of Medicine and Dentistry of New Jersey, 150 Bergen Street, G-142, Newark, NJ 07103, USA
E-mail address: wallacgf@umdnj.edu

Clin Podiatr Med Surg 27 (2010) 407–416
doi:10.1016/j.cpm.2010.04.002
0891-8422/10/$ – see front matter © 2010 Elsevier Inc. All rights reserved.

podiatric.theclinics.com

A : Aggravated

What aggravated the lesion; certain shoes, activities, treatments?

T : Treatment

What previous treatment(s) have been tried (whether over the counter, from another physician, or a home remedy)?

PLANTAR VERRUCA

The human papilloma virus (HPV1,2,4) causes plantar verruca.[1] The presentation can be as a solitary lesion or grouped, the mosaic variety. Both can be difficult to eradicate.

The patient may provide a history of walking barefoot or stepping on a piece of glass or other foreign body that, although removed, still feels as though something is there. A careful examination should dispel any presence of a foreign body. Other and more common histories just deal with an idiopathic presentation.

A verruca usually, but not always, will present with the following characteristics: loss of skin lines through the lesion, dolor on lateral compression of the verruca, capillary buds that freely bleed on debridement, and a fibrous, cauliflowerlike texture.[2] One should not wait to see any capillary buds or bleeding to make the diagnosis. Some exhibit no discernable buds or never bleed on debridement. As a result of ambulation, the verruca may be flush with the skin and not raised. On the rims of the heel the lesion will be elevated. The mosaic variety shows multiple areas of coalesced verrucae and appears more dessicated than the single verruca. Both patterns can coexist. Multiple areas on the heel and foot can be affected.

The contralateral foot and hands should be inspected for additional lesions. A time line should be established, especially when multiple areas are affected or more than 1 verruca is present. For example, how long ago did the first one and the last one appear? Treatment is problematic when new lesions are appearing rapidly. Another important consideration is the presence or absence of hyperhidrosis. Walling[3] found a significant increase in verrucae in the presence of hyperhidrosis. The hyperhidrosis must be addressed simultaneously with any verruca treatment.

There are many treatments for verruca eradication.[4–6] No treatment stands out as a panacea. At University Hospital, University of Medicine and Dentistry of New Jersey (UMDNJ), the protocol is to treat the lesion conservatively, according to the individual clinician's preference, although most use some form of salicylic acid. After 12 weeks without success, the patient undergoes blunt dissection in the manner of Pringle and Helms.[7] After excision in toto of the verruca, the base is cauterized with phenol. Gelfoam, an antibiotic ointment, and a compressive dressing are applied. The patient is instructed to remove same in 24 hours and begin twice-daily Epsom salt soaks followed by the application of an antibiotic ointment and a dressing. The first visit is in 1 week. The laser is used for multiple lesions. Three important caveats are noted when performing blunt dissection: (1) any specimen is sent for pathologic analysis. This policy is especially relevant for physicians who use laser ablation of verrucae. Before lasering the verruca, a piece should be obtained and sent to pathology. (2) The entire lesion is excised encompassing a few millimeters beyond the visible borders. (3) The superficial fascia is not violated. There should never be adipose tissue in the surgical site; this would mean that the excision was too deep and raises the possibility of the formation of a prominent scar. The potential for a plantar scar is what generates criticism for surgical excision.[5]

Gibbs and colleagues[8] provided a systematic review of multiple therapies; however, they do not mention surgical means for excision. The evidence from the literature did support using salicylic acid.

The person who is immunocompromised, especially with human immunodeficiency virus (HIV)/acquired immune deficiency syndrome (AIDS), poses a unique challenge for cure regardless of the type of treatment selected. Patients with the HIV virus had a greater surface area infected with verrucae and exhibited an increased recurrence rate after treatment, even if surgery was performed.[9] Education will be beneficial to these patients to provide realistic outcomes.

Verrucae have a great potential for recurrence.[10] Logical suggestions are to keep the feet dry; rotate shoes; avoid being barefoot, especially in public areas; and report sighting new lesions as soon as possible.

XEROSIS AND FISSURES

Xerosis of the foot may be confined to the heel, especially the rims, but more likely will encompass the entire foot. If just at the heel rims, this can progress to hyperkeratosis and eventually fissures.

Xerosis is usually caused by a loss of skin hydration, and is more pronounced in dry and low humidity climates. Advanced age is a also predisposing factor. The elastin and collagen content of the skin are decreased with aging.[11] An emollient with urea is a good initial treatment. In milder cases, an emollient used on the hands can be applied to the feet. There are prescription products available for more severe cases.

Hyperkeratotic lesions on the rims of the calcaneus are usually caused by shoes being worn without a heel counter.[12] The normal calcaneal movement during gait is not held firmly by any heel counter and the body reacts with the hyperkeratosis. Often, relief can only be obtained after debridement. Shoes with heel counters and applying an emollient can mitigate or eliminate the skin pathology. The emollient's efficacy can be enhanced by applying under occlusion (eg, Saran Wrap). Any medication should be applied liberally, and preferably after a shower or bath (**Fig. 1**).

Should the hyperkeratosis or xerosis become thickened, the development of fissures is more likely (**Fig. 2**). Pain can be present to a greater degree with fissures. If the fissures penetrate beyond the epidermis, bleeding can ensue. Cellulitis will then be a possibility, and should be treated appropriately. Treatment is the same as for hyperkeratosis, with the possible addition of topical antibiotic or systemic agents if cellulitic. Fissures and cellulitis in a patient with diabetes are causes for alarm.[13]

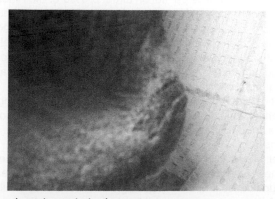

Fig. 1. Xerosis of heel causing pain in shoes.

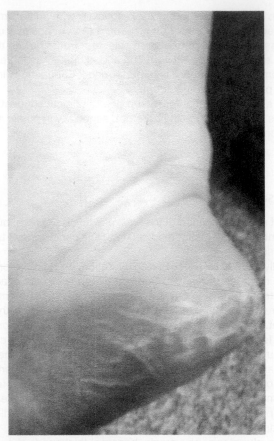

Fig. 2. Superficial fissures evident on heels.

IPK

An IPK is probably the most common plantar lesion encountered on the plantar surface of the foot. These lesions appear on weight-bearing surfaces.

Unlike a verruca, the IPK will be painful on direct pressure. Skin lines run through the lesion. The center is composed of keratin and surrounded by a cornuted lamella.[14,15] Debridement will eliminate the pain until recurrence. Radiographs should be obtained to determine whether there is an underlying exostosis. A calcaneal axial should be included with the 3 standard views. Removal of the osseous pathology can eliminate the IPK. Underlying hardware, especially if backing out, can lead to an IPK. Hardware and lesion removal most likely will solve the problem.

In most instances there is no bony causal agent. Although debriding the IPK relieves symptoms, the effect is only temporary in most instances. Various conservative modalities can be tried, with none providing a sure remedy.[16,17] Blunt dissection can also be attempted.

An IPK is a focal, almost pinpoint, lesion. A callus or tyloma or hyperkeratosis lesion is more diffuse. These appear secondary to abnormal pressure. There may be a biomechanical or structural cause. For example, a rigid cavus foot may exhibit a callus on the plantar surface of the calcaneus in addition to those beneath metatarsals 1 and 5 (tripod). Hyperkeratoses may be on the lateral rim of the calcaneus secondary to rear-foot/calcaneal varus. Debridement may provide relief. Surgical correction of osseous deformities may lead to elimination.

DERMAL ATROPHY

Plantar fasciitis is discussed in the article by Healey and Chen elsewhere in this issue. Injections of corticosteroids into the heel are a common treatment modality. One of the complications of these steroid injections is dermal atrophy.[18] Loss of dermal content can potentially lead to heel pain. Therefore, the timing and number of corticosteroid injections need to be kept to a minimum. There is no consensus regarding the frequency and number of injections that can be administered into the heel, whether in the same location or in more widespread areas. At UMDNJ the rubric followed is no more than 3 injections in 6 months. The first sign of dermal atrophy results in the cessation of any further injections.

Aging can also lead to dermal atrophy. The entire heel lacks resiliency and fat-pad cushioning. The calcaneus then becomes more prominent when ambulating with not only pain but the potential increase of epidermal lesions. Combined with xerosis of aging, there is a need for an agent to decrease the xerosis and another to cushion the heel.

Clemow and colleagues[19] grouped the causal factors of aging and steroid injections into a category called fat-pad syndrome. There is likely to be visible thinning of the plantar heel fat pad. The patient will complain of a more diffuse pain in the heel. The plantar fascia would not be symptomatic. Treatment is supportive and relies on cushioning of the heel.

Even diabetic heels exhibit diminished cushioning. Macro- and microchambers found in the soft tissue of the heel are normally heterogeneous. In patients with diabetes, the macrochambers have increased stiffness, whereas microchambers have a decrease in stiffness. The resiliency of the heel fat pad is ultimately compromised. Any reduction in cushioning can lead to tissue breakdown.[20] This is especially significant when accompanied by diabetic neuropathy.

A calcaneal fracture can disrupt the septae around the heel, especially when caused by a fall from a height (**Fig. 3**).[21,22] Dermal atrophy may be the visible evidence of this disruption. However, the patient may continue to have heel pain even though there is no discernable atrophy. Nothing may manifest until the patient begins ambulation.

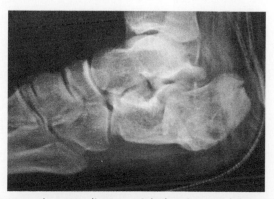

Fig. 3. Calcaneal fracture that may disrupt weight-bearing capabilities.

The septal architecture can never be reestablished. Accommodative devices can be tried in the hope of providing some relief.

Calcaneal fractures may present with ecchymosis within the arch and extending proximally. This condition is referred to as Mondor sign and is pathognomonic for calcaneal fractures (see earlier discussion). Although this finding is not painful in itself, there will be pain from the calcaneal fracture. It is included here as an important dermatologic finding in a diagnosis causing pain. Discoloration is plantar, even encompassing the soft tissue of the heel itself.

FRICTION BLISTERS

Blisters can form on the heel and rims, usually as a result of abnormal, rapid motion, such as playing basketball. They can be painful.

A blister is a separation of the epidermis from the dermis and is usually filled with serous fluid. Occasionally, serosaginous fluid appears. The contents are sterile.[23]

Treatment consists of puncturing the sides of the blister, extravasating the fluid, and allowing the roof to collapse and serve as a biologic dressing. An antibiotic and non-adherent dressing can be applied until healed. In people with diabetes, the roof is removed with the same treatment.

The patient will occasionally remove the roof, or the roof will slough on its own. These patients have pain until the base of the blister toughens. Care is supportive, consisting of an antibiotic and nonadherent dressing.

The patient may want to continue engaging in the sports or running that caused the blister. Prevention of blisters should begin with an inspection of the shoes for any worn areas or decrease in shock absorption. If these are present, then the shoes must be replaced. The old standbys of wearing 2 pairs of socks and applying an emollient before initiating the sporting activity may be prophylactic for blister formation.

OTHER DERMATOLOGIC CAUSES OF HEEL PAIN

Heel ulcers can have many causes. The 2 most common are neuropathy in a patient with diabetes, and abnormal pressure; a decubitus ulcer. In addition, Achilles lengthening can create a calcaneal gait and can lead to an ulcer in the patient with neuropathy.[24] The amount of ischemia or neuropathy will lead to a range of pain from none to possible intense pain (**Fig. 4**).

In all instances, the calcaneus is evaluated for osteomyelitis. Any ulcer on the heel undergoes the following: (1) etiologic discovery, (2) diagnostic workup, (3) debridement,

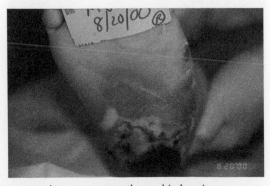

Fig. 4. Diabetic ulcer secondary to neuropathy and ischemia.

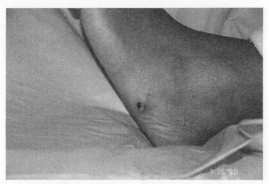

Fig. 5. Lesion on lateral border of heel. Incisional biopsy was positive for melanoma, necessitating wide excision.

(4) topical treatment, (5) surgical treatment if indicated, (6) off-loading, and (7) appropriate antibiotic coverage.[25–27]

Although contact dermatitis, psoriasis, and tinea pedis may not present with pain per se, they can be present on the heels. A thorough history and examination can differentiate them. A biopsy of any lesion, especially when treatment fails, can provide an accurate diagnosis. Results of the biopsy will dictate treatment.

Box 1
Soft-tissue masses presenting on the heel

Pyogenic granuloma

Rheumatoid nodule

Lipoma

Inclusion cyst

Eccrine poroma

Fibroma

Malignant soft-tissue masses

Bulla

Fracture blisters

Tophae

Ganglion

Xanthoma

Nevus

Basal, squamous cell carcinomas

Melanoma

Neuroma

Piezogenic papules

Miscellaneous

Cicatrix

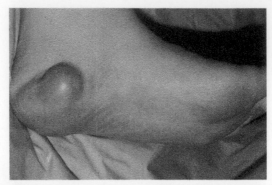

Fig. 6. Excision of soft-tissue mass encompassing plantar and medial aspects of heel yielded rheumatoid nodule.

Various malignant skin tumors can appear on the heel. The more common are basal and squamous cell carcinomas and melanomas. The latter is the most lethal. Pain may not be present. An index of suspicion is raised when any unusual lesion is present (**Fig. 5**). A biopsy will confirm the diagnosis. Results of the biopsy will dictate treatment.

Underlying soft-tissue masses, benign or malignant, may cause heel pain. In most cases, the pain is caused by ambulation/pressure on the mass and not necessarily by the mass itself. Any presentation of a soft-tissue mass needs to be evaluated further. The routine use of aspiration should be discouraged, especially before any workup. Aspiration for cytopathological analysis can be used for some tumors.[28] **Box 1** lists some soft-tissue masses that may appear on the heel (**Fig. 6**).

A cicatrix may be painful. Usually it is painful because the scar is not fine lined or there is entrapment of nerve tissue. The former can be mitigated with meticulous surgical technique and a period of non–weight bearing immediately after surgery until the sutures are removed, usually at 3 weeks. The latter may exhibit a Tinel sign on palpation. Topical agents can be tried for both. Surgical excision may have to be performed to eradicate the symptoms. An additional cause may be prominent internal fixation or screw loosening. In either case, they are removed after osseous healing.

Any dermatologic condition can affect the calcaneus. These most likely will not just be segregated to the heel but will appear on the rest of the foot. Dermatologic presentations require the examination of hands and feet. The possibility of examining other parts of the body cannot be excluded. Never rule out a dermatology consultation.

Other diagnoses appearing on the heel, although in many cases not symptomatic, are talon noir, pitted keratolysis, various genokeratoses, hyperhidrosis, dyshidrosis, and cold injury.

SUMMARY

Heel pain can be multifactoral. The cause of the pain may be a dermatologic entity. The foot and ankle surgeon has to keep in mind that various skin conditions can cause heel pain.

REFERENCES

1. Landsman MJ, Mancuso JE, Abramow SP. Diagnosis, pathophysiology, and treatment of plantar verruca. Clin Podiatr Med Surg 1996;13(1):55–71.

2. Dockery GL. Viral skin infections. In: Cutaneous disorders of the lower extremity. Philadelphia: WB Saunders; 1997. p. 67–82.
3. Walling HW. Primary hyperhidrosis increases the risk of cutaneous infection: a case-control study of 387 patients. J Am Acad Dermatol 2009;61(2):242–6.
4. Jennings MB, Ricketti J, Guadara J, et al. Treatment for simple plantar verrucae: monochloroacetic acid and 10% formaldehyde versus 10% formaldehyde alone. J Am Podiatr Med Assoc 2006;96(1):53–8.
5. Lipke MM. An armamentarium of wart treatments. Clin Med Res 2006;4(4): 273–93.
6. Park HS, Choi WS. Pulsed dye laser treatment for viral warts: a study of 120 patients. J Dermatol 2008;35(8):491–8.
7. Pringle WM, Helms DC. Treatment of plantar warts by blunt dissection. Arch Dermatol 1973;108(1):79–82.
8. Gibbs S, Harvey I, Sterling J, et al. Local treatment for cutaneous warts: systematic review. BMJ 2002;325(7362):461–4.
9. Whitaker JM, Gaggero GI, Loveland L, et al. Plantar verrucae in patients with human immunodeficiency virus. Clinical presentation and treatment response. J Am Podiatr Med Assoc 2001;91(2):79–84.
10. Pieacher MD, Dexter WW. Cutaneous fungal and viral infections in athletes. Clin Sports Med 2007;26:397–411.
11. Farage MA, Miller KW, Berardesca E, et al. Clinical implications of aging skin: cutaneous disorders in the elderly. Am J Clin Dermatol 2009;10(2):73–86.
12. Fuller EA. A review of the biomechanics of shoes. Clin Podiatr Med Surg 1994; 11(2):241–58.
13. Frykberg RG, Zgonis T, Armstrong DG, et al. Diabetic foot disorders: a clinical practice guideline. J Foot Ankle Surg 2006;45(55):S1–S66.
14. Kress DW. Dermatology of the foot and lower extremity. In: Coughlin MJ, Mann RA, Saltzman CL, editors. Surgery of the foot and ankle. Philadelphia: Mosby; 2007. p. 1809–23.
15. McCarthy DJ. Dermatologic and soft tissue disorders. In: Levy LA, Hetherington VJ, editors. Principles and practice of podiatric medicine. New York: Churchill Livingstone; 1990. p. 465–98.
16. Balkin SW. Injectable silicone and the foot: a 41-year clinical and histologic history. Dermatol Surg 2005;31(11):1555–9.
17. Silfverskiold JP. Common foot problems: relieving the pain of bunions, keratoses, corns, and calluses. Postgrad Med 1991;89(5):183–8.
18. Salerno A, Heiniann R. Efficacy and safety of steroid use for postoperative pain relief. J Bone Joint Surg Am 2006;88(6):1361–71.
19. Clemow C, Pope B, Woodall HE. Tools to speed your heel pain diagnosis. J Fam Pract 2008;57(11):714–22.
20. Chih-Chin H, Wen-Chung T, Tzu-Yo H, et al. Diabetic effects on microchambers and macrochambers tissue properties in human heel pads. Clin Biomech 2009; 24:682–6.
21. Lim EVA, Leung JPF. Complications of intraarticular calcaneal fractures. Clin Orthop Relat Res 2001;391:7–16.
22. Sanders R. Displaced intra-articular fractures of the calcaneus. J Bone Joint Surg Am 2000;82(2):225–50.
23. Knapik JJ, Reynolds KL, Duplantis KL, et al. Friction blisters: pathophysiology, prevention and treatment. Sports Med 1995;20(3):136–47.
24. Chilvers M, Malicky ES, Anderson TG, et al. Heel overload associated with heel cord insufficiency. Foot Ankle Int 2007;28(6):687–9.

25. Brooks KR, Abidi NA, Vieira P. Calcanectomy for treatment of the infected os calcis. Tech Foot Ankle Surg 2004;3:165–76.
26. Suess JS, Kim PJ, Steinberg JS. Negative pressure wound therapy: evidence-
based treatment for complex diabetic wounds. Curr Diab Rep 2006;6:446–50.
27. Steinberg JS, Werber B, Kim PJ. Bioengineered alternative tissues for the
surgical management of diabetic foot ulceration. In: Zgonis T, editor. Surgical
reconstruction of the diabetic foot and ankle. Philadelphia: Worters Kluwer;
2009. p. 100–18.
28. Wakely PE Jr, Kneisl JS. Soft tissue aspiration cytopathology. Cancer 2000;90(5):
292–8.

Management of Calcaneal Osteomyelitis

Katherine Chen, DPM[a],*, Rachel Balloch, DPM, AACFAS[b]

KEYWORDS

• Calcaneal osteomyelitis • Debridement • Foot

Osteomyelitis comes from the Greek words "osteon" for bone and "myelo" for marrow. Auguste Nelaton, a surgeon from Paris, first coined the term osteomyelitis in 1844 to describe a localized bone and marrow infection.[1] Osteomyelitis of the calcaneus presents foot-and-ankle surgeons with a complicated situation that requires careful planning and thorough evaluation. The difficulty lies in that the calcaneus is on a weight bearing surface, where there is often poor tissue coverage to close the wound and anatomically the vascularity of the skin envelope is poor. Therefore, quick and accurate diagnosis is essential to save both limb and life.

There are several classifications of osteomyelitis. In 1970, Waldvogel classified osteomyelitis based on the different routes of infection.[2]

1. Hematogenous
2. Direct or contiguous infection
   No vascular disease present
   Vascular disease present
3. Chronic.

Hematogenous osteomyelitis is usually caused by bacterial seeding from the blood. It is more common in children because of the highly vascularized metaphysis of growing bones; however, it can be seen in patients of all ages. Osteomyelitis of the calcaneus is usually seen in the posterior aspect adjacent to the apophysis.[3] It is thought that in the long bones of children there is a lack of phagocytic lining cells in the afferent metaphyseal loops of long bone as well as inactive phagocytic lining cells in the efferent metaphyseal loops. Trueta[4] explains the different types of metaphyseal vascular supply depending on the age of the person. In infants and children younger than 1 year, vessels penetrate the epiphyseal growth plate to supply the epiphysis.

---

[a] University Hospital, University of Medicine and Dentistry of New Jersey, 150 Bergen Street, G-142, Newark, NJ 07103, USA
[b] 162 Mansfield Avenue, Willimantic, CT 06226, USA
* Corresponding author.
E-mail address: chenk2@umdnj.edu

Clin Podiatr Med Surg 27 (2010) 417–429
doi:10.1016/j.cpm.2010.04.003
0891-8422/10/$ – see front matter. Published by Elsevier Inc.

podiatric.theclinics.com

Therefore, infections can cross the growth plate and infect joint spaces. This spread can lead to early closure of the growth plate. In children older than 1 year, vessels do not penetrate the growth plate. Hence, the plate acts as a barrier preventing infections from entering the epiphysis and ultimately the joints.

Direct or contiguous osteomyelitis is caused by contact of the tissue and bacteria or continuous spread from an adjacent source. This method of inoculation can typically occur after surgery, with ulcerations, open fractures, or penetrating wounds in the foot. Clinical manifestations are more localized when compared with hematogenous osteomyelitis.

The vascular status of the patient can play an important role in causing direct calcaneal osteomyelitis. Vascular insufficiency can lead to soft tissue necrosis and decreased healing capacities once the skin is broken or the bone is exposed. On the other hand, individuals can have patent vessels and still have chronic decubital ulcerations, if they are bedridden.

Chronic osteomyelitis is seen in bone infections that have been present for long periods of time with persistence of microorganisms and that have received inadequate treatment. Wounds that fail to heal or intermittently reopen are more prone to chronic osteomyelitis. At this stage, surgical debridement is necessary to eradicate the infection because antibiotic treatment alone would not be sufficient.

In 1985, Cierny and colleagues[5] introduced a classification that was based on the anatomic extent of the infection through the bone and the health of the host. This is known as the Cierny-Mader classification that first divides the osseous anatomy into

1. Medullary only
2. Superficial cortex
3. Localized
4. Diffuse.

Then the classification separates the patients into 3 groups:

1. Healthy patients
2. Compromised patients (local compromise, systemic compromise)
3. Patients who were not candidates for surgery because the treatment was worse than the disease.

In 1984, Kelly[6] devised a classification for adult osteomyelitis and its relationship to fracture healing. This classification differentiated osteomyelitis into hematogenous, associated with a fracture with union, associated with a fracture with nonunion, or a postoperative wound without fracture.

ETIOLOGY

Osteomyelitis of the calcaneus can be seen in a variety of clinical situations. Soft tissue infections, decubital and diabetic ulcers, penetrating wounds, crush injuries, and open fractures may extend and destroy the bone adjacent to it. Patients with rheumatoid arthritis, vasculitis, and leukopenia and those on corticosteroid and/or immunosuppressant therapy are also at risk for developing bone infections. Puncture wounds can but rarely become osteomyelitic, with an incidence rate of 1.8% in the pediatric population.[7]

Once a microorganism infiltrates into the heel, the inflammatory factors and leukocytes contribute to tissue necrosis and destruction of bone trabeculae and bone matrix. Vascular channels are compressed and obliterated, which progress to ischemia and bone necrosis.[2] Avascular bone can then separate and harbor bacteria.

Gram-positive cocci are the most common causative organism of calcaneal osteomyelitis. *Staphylococcus aureus*, *Staphylococcus epidermidis*, and *Streptococcus* spp account for 73% of osteomyelitis after surgical procedures.[8] In patients younger than 2 years, hematogenous osteomyelitis is commonly caused by Haemophilus influenza, whereas in adults, S aureus is the primary causative organism. Pseudomonas aeruginosa is common in traumatic injury–related osteomyelitis. Anaerobic, gram-negative, or mixed gram-positive and gram-negative infections are the usual causes of diabetic or vascular compromised osteomyelitis.

The prevalence of methicillin-resistant S aureus (MRSA) has shifted treatment paradigms for patients with calcaneal osteomyelitis. The antibiotic of choice is different if the patient has MRSA rather than methicillin-susceptible S aureus due to increased drug resistance. MRSA can be further divided into community acquired and hospital acquired. The differentiation is based more on the clinical onset than on antibiotic resistance. Community-acquired MRSA is seen in patients who have had no recent hospitalization, surgery, dialysis, indwelling catheter, or previous MRSA infection.[9] These patients often have an infection that is present or diagnosed within 48 to 72 hours of admission. Hospital-acquired MRSA is seen in patients who entered the hospital without an MRSA infection and later developed one while hospitalized. One should be suspicious of MRSA infection, if their community is known to have increased numbers of MRSA infections or if the patient is not responding to antibiotics that do not cover MRSA.

Laughlin and colleagues[10] performed a prospective study in Texas of all patients with calcaneal osteomyelitis from 1984 to 1993 to determine if there was a correlation between etiology, host, and pathogen. The number of gram-positive organisms was comparable in patients independent of host classification. A compromised host was found to have more gram-negative and anaerobic organisms. Patients who had problems with sensation in the foot, such as diabetic patients and patients with cranial nerve lesions, were also noticed to have in addition an anaerobic organism cultured.

SYMPTOMS

Hematogenous calcaneal osteomyelitis accounts for 3% to 10% of acute pediatric bony infections.[9] It peaks in children younger than 3 years and again between 7 and 9 years. Hematogenous osteomyelitis usually manifests only after having bacteremia. Children present with abrupt onset of pain, tenderness, and systemic symptoms of infection such as fever, chills, and malaise. On physical examination, erythema, tenderness in the ankle or foot, warmth, and edema are noted. Secondary to pain, toe walking or inability to bear weight to the heel is seen during gait analysis. Some children lay with the heel up by hanging the affected leg over the other leg to prevent the foot from touching the bed and causing pain.

Contiguous osteomyelitis should be suspected if there is a nonhealing ulcer, sinus tract, drainage, or fluctuance. It can be seen in patients of all ages, with chronic ulcerations, previous lacerations, puncture wounds, open trauma, or postoperatively. The patient presents with pain, stiffness, mild-to-moderate swelling, and erythema of the affected area. A positive probe-to-bone test should obviate a need for further evaluation such as radiography, magnetic resonance imaging (MRI), or bone biopsy.

According to Jaakkola and Kehl,[11] an average of 13.1 days pass before calcaneal osteomyelitis begins to show symptoms. Any index of suspicion should be followed up to prevent further infectious damage to the calcaneus.

DIAGNOSIS

Leukocytosis may or may not be present and should not be used as an absolute indicator of osteomyelitis. In the acute stage, elevation of the white blood cell count may be seen. However, this condition is not true in all patients. In a study by Armstrong and colleagues,[12] 54% of the patients with acute osteomyelitis presented with normal white blood cell count. This condition is especially seen in diabetic patients. Once the infectious process becomes chronic, the white blood cell count may also be normal, leading some physicians to believe that no infection exists.

Other laboratory tests can also help determine if an infection is present. Erythrocyte sedimentation rate is a nonspecific marker for inflammation. A result greater than 70 mm/h increases the likelihood of osteomyelitis. This test gives a sensitivity of 89.5% and a specificity of 100% for osteomyelitis.[13] C-reactive protein is another nonspecific marker produced by the liver during acute stages of inflammation. It may be more useful than the erythrocyte sedimentation rate because it shows an elevation earlier. Once treatment is started, C-reactive protein levels also quickly decrease. If clinical symptoms exist but no elevation in either marker is present, osteomyelitis cannot be ruled out.

Probe to bone is a test that throughout the years has grown out of favor as an absolute indicator for osteomyelitis. Grayson and colleagues[14] found that the sensitivity of a positive probe-to-bone test was 66% and the specificity was 85%. Lavery and colleagues[15] found a positive predictive value of 57% to 62% with a negative predictive value of 96% to 98% for osteomyelitis in foot wounds of diabetic patients. The rule of thumb is if the bone is palpable, one should be suspicious for associated osteomyelitis because it means the bacteria is capable of coming in contact with the bone.

Cultures should be taken if a draining sinus tract is present. Bacteria can create a glycocalyx film over the wound, which makes them inaccessible to culture. Therefore, before taking any culture, curettage or debridement of the wound should be performed to make identification more accurate. Mackowiak and colleagues[16] revealed that cultures obtained from draining sinus tracts and soft tissue specimens next to the suspect bone infection fail to identify the causative organism. In their study, 102 cultures out of 183 taken from 35 patients were noted to be different from operative cultures. The only organism that was correctly identified most of the time was Staphylococcus from monomicrobial infections. According to Lavery and colleagues,[17] only 36% of soft tissue cultures accurately identify the organisms in diabetic patients. On the other hand, serial tissue cultures have been able to better isolate the organisms, if the same organism is persistently present.

The gold standard for diagnosing osteomyelitis is taking a bone biopsy, which is sent for both microbiologic and pathologic examination. The location of the biopsy should not be taken through the sinus tract. A separate incision should be made in order not to contaminate the result with bacteria from the soft tissue. Biopsies are taken with a Jamshidi self-contained bone marrow needle, which consists of an outer cannula and a handle with an inner stylet for tissue penetration. The needle is directed at the calcaneus and the bone is aspirated. The wound can then be closed primarily, if needed. Patients should not be treated with antibiotics before performing a bone biopsy. Bacterial growth can be suppressed when the patient is on antibiotics, which interferes with proper identification of the organism. If the patient is already on antibiotics, treatment should be stopped for a minimum of 48 hours before performing the bone biopsy.

DIAGNOSTIC MODALITIES

Osteomyelitic findings on plain radiographs lag approximately 2 weeks behind the process of the infection. About 30% to 60% of bone demineralizes before radiographic evidence is noted. The mean sensitivity of radiography is 67% and the mean specificity is 40% in diagnosing osteomyelitis.[18] If no radiographic evidence is present, but clinical suspicion is high, other forms of diagnostic studies should be considered.

In the acute phase, soft tissue swelling and obliteration of fascial planes may be the only radiographic signs. Sometimes, radiographs may demonstrate subperiosteal new bone formation and/or localized loss of bone density. As time progresses and the osteomyelitis becomes subacute, well-defined lytic lesions with sclerotic rims, otherwise known as Brodie abscess, can be seen. In chronic stages of osteomyelitis, sequestra (devascularized dead bone), involucrum (new bone formation laid over dead bone), and cloaca (opening in the cortex for purulence to drain through) can be seen.

Ultrasonography demonstrates changes as early as 1 to 2 days after onset of symptoms. It shows abnormalities including soft tissue abscess, fluid collections, and periosteal elevation. However, it does not allow for visualization of the calcaneal cortex.

Many different types of bone scintigraphy are available to diagnose osteomyelitis. They can identify osteomyelitis as early as 24 to 48 hours after the onset of the infection. However, the scans may create false-positive results if the patient has cellulitis, osteoarthropathy, open epiphysis, experienced recent trauma, or underwent surgery. Once the infection becomes chronic, it no longer shows increased uptake. Technetium Tc 99m bone scan has a mean sensitivity of 85% and mean specificity of 54%.[19] It demonstrates osteoblastic absorption on the surfaces of hydroxyapatite crystals and accumulates in areas of increased periosteal, endosteal, or osseous vascularity and physiologic activity. This scan is more beneficial as a screening process to determine the presence or absence of bone disease (**Fig. 1**). Gallium Ga 67 citrate scan is performed 24 to 48 hours after infection. Gallium Ga 67 citrate is thought to bind to white blood cells, plasma proteins, transferrin, ferritin, lactoferrin, and siderophores that travel to areas of inflammation. The sensitivity is 81% with a specificity of 29%.[20] Indium In 111 oxine binds to cytoplasmic components of white blood cell membranes. Leukocytes are isolated from venous blood and labeled with Indium In 111 oxine and injected into the patient. After 24 hours, the patient is scanned. Sensitivity and specificity is 100% and 70%, respectively.[21]

Computed tomography (CT) is a useful tool to determine the severity of the soft tissue infection as well as the extent of bony destruction. It is 66% sensitive in detecting osteomyelitis and 52% sensitive in detecting abscess.[22] Cortical destruction, periosteal proliferation, and soft tissue extension can be seen well on CT images.

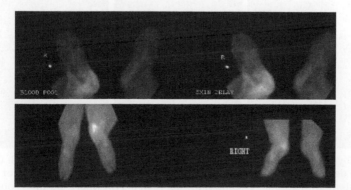

Fig. 1. A 51-year-old diabetic male with chronic heel ulceration. Three-phase bone scan demonstrate increased uptake in the right heel consistent with calcaneal osteomyelitis along the posteroinferior aspect of the calcaneus.

Emphysema and fluid collections such as abscesses and sinus tracts in soft tissue and bone can also be seen.

MRI has a high sensitivity and a high specificity of 94% and 85.5%, respectively, for detecting osteomyelitis. It is 97% sensitive in diagnosing an abscess.[22] On a T1-weighted sequence, there Is abnormal marrow with low signal intensity, whereas on T2, there is high signal intensity. Marrow signal abnormalities can be reliably noted on an MR image. Bone destruction and soft tissue abnormalities such as overlying ulcerations, cellulitis, phlegmon, abscess, and sinus tracts can be visualized (**Figs. 2** and **3**).

TREATMENTS

Calcaneal osteomyelitis is a difficult condition to treat. Often, the osteomyelitis is associated with some sort of ulceration, which makes tissue coverage challenging. Treatments include antibiotic therapy, debridement, partial or total calcanectomy, flap coverage, and below-knee amputations. Therapeutic choice is sometimes patient driven, surgeon's choice, or the only option secondary to the availability of soft tissue coverage and/or vascular status of the patient. Ideally, for a salvage procedure to succeed, the ankle-brachial index should be greater than 0.45, transcutaneous Po_2 greater than 28 mm Hg, and albumin level greater than 3.0 g/dL.[8] The albumin level, along with transferrin level represents the nutritional status of the patient. If any of the abovementioned parameters are suboptimal, an appropriate consultation is required.

Before accessibility of wound and bone cultures results, the patient should be placed on empiric parenteral antibiotics. Once the culture sensitivities are available, number of antimicrobials should be changed to one or more specific to the bacteria and the minimum inhibitory concentrations. The length of antibiotic treatment can be anywhere from 4 to 6 weeks. If the antibiotic therapy is adequate, further destruction of bone and soft tissue should be arrested. Patients at this point can go home with oral antibiotics for continued therapy. Children should receive 2 weeks of initial parenteral antibiotic therapy before changing to an oral antibiotic for the remaining period of treatment.[23] If the infectious process becomes a chronic condition, antibiotics alone may not be sufficient.

Surgical incision and drainage is performed to remove any necrotic soft tissue and bone. It can decompress abscesses by removing any pockets of infection. Gas in the

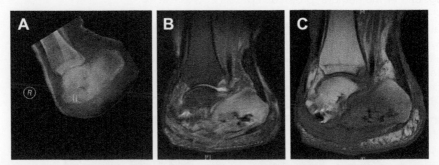

Fig. 2. A 70-year-old diabetic male with a chronic ulceration of the right heel. (*A*) Lateral radiograph demonstrating patchy sclerosis and erosions of the plantar aspect of the calcaneus consistent with chronic osteomyelitis. (*B, C*) MRI STIR (short tau inversion recovery) image and T1-weighted image, respectively, reveal diffuse bone marrow edema throughout the calcaneus with areas of low signal intensity within the calcaneal body and posterior process consistent with gas.

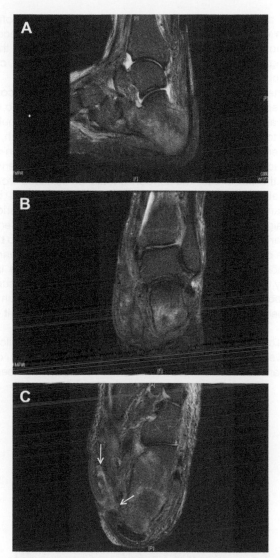

Fig. 3. A 65-year-old diabetic male admitted for septic shock presenting with ulceration plantar heel. (*A, B*) MRI STIR (short tau inversion recovery) image with increased signal intensity at the posterior aspect of the calcaneus. (*C*) Abscess along the medial aspect of the ankle.

tissue represents a surgical emergency. Debridement of bone should be performed until raw bleeding is noted. If internal fixation or prostheses are present, their stability should be determined. Any loosening of hardware should be corrected by removing the fixation and converting to external fixation, if necessary. If the hardware is stable, it should be left in.

Antibiotic-impregnated polymethylmethacrylate (PMMA) beads are used to fill any bone defects, maintain bony contours, and maximize density while also managing the osteomyelitis. Antibiotics capable of being mixed with the PMMA beads are gentamycin, vancomycin, tobramycin, or clindamycin. Through this modality, high concentration of antibiotics can be delivered to the bone and soft tissue without increasing serum concentrations to toxic levels. It is generally recommended that the beads be removed no later than 14 to 17 days after implantation through a second procedure. Biodegradable antibiotic beads, such as calcium sulfate, can remain in the surgical site without removal.

A partial calcanectomy is an option for treating a heel ulcer with concomitant osteomyelitis. The vascular status of the patient should be evaluated to determine if the patient has the capacity to heal the wound. Surgical incisions should be planned if the ulcer is going to be excised too. If the ulcer is 7 cm or less in width, primary closure of the wound after partial calcanectomy is possible.[24] The incision should be large enough to allow access to the posterior calcaneus. If the Achilles tendon is impeding the resection of the calcaneus, the tendon should be released from the posterior aspect of the calcaneus. Any necrotic exposed tendon should be debrided or resected. The plantar fascia should also be released from the inferior aspect of the calcaneus. A straight osteotome or sagittal saw is then used to resect the calcaneus from posterosuperior to antero-inferior position, starting posterior to the subtalar joint and ending at the calcaneocuboid joint, although these points can vary depending on the amount of bone that needs to be resected. If indicated, the incision may be extended laterally to resect more of the bone to properly close the surgical site. Postoperatively, the foot should be splinted in plantar flexion for a minimum of 4 to 6 weeks to allow for proper healing of the skin and the Achilles tendon, if it was transected (**Fig. 4**).

Bollinger and Thordarson[24] studied 22 patients with large heel ulcerations with or without osteomyelitis of the calcaneus and performed partial calcanectomies. Improvement in ambulation and pain status was reviewed. Eighteen patients were

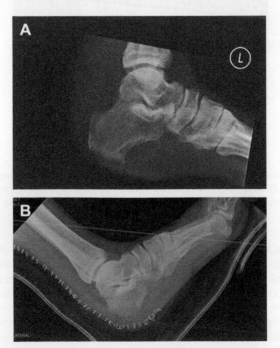

Fig. 4. (A) Preoperative calcaneus with plantar heel ulcer. (B) Partial calcanectomy after serial debridements and antibiotics for 6 months.

available for follow-up. Twelve had delayed wound healing that required either a split-thickness skin graft or serial debridements. Postoperative ambulatory status improved in 7 patients, did not change in 10 patients, and decreased in 1 patient. After the partial calcanectomy, 6 patients reported no pain, 10 had mild pain, 1 had moderate pain, and 1 had severe pain. They found that the use of this procedure prevented the immediate need for a below-knee amputation in patients with large heel ulcers and osteomyelitis of the calcaneus.

Total calcanectomy is a good alternative to a below-knee amputation. This procedure can be used if partial calcanectomy fails or if the heel ulcer is greater than 50% of the heel pad.[25] It allows for total eradication of the infection by removing the source and still preserves ambulation. A Gaenslen "heel splitting" curvilinear incision is made starting at the Achilles tendon and extending either medially or laterally. The incision is straight to the bone, and the soft tissue around the calcaneus is freed.

Patients who undergo a partial or total calcanectomy can be placed in a custom-molded heel containment orthosis and an ankle-foot orthosis to reduce the shear force upon the soft tissue around the heel and also to redistribute weight.

Soft tissue coverage after debridement can become an issue if the foot is not amenable to closure. Split-thickness skin grafts can be an option to cover the defect, but the forces of weight bearing on the heel can lead to failure of the graft.[26]

The use of a fasciocutaneous flap was first described by Pontén[27] in 1981 to repair soft tissue defects of the lower leg. Muscle and myocutaneous flaps are rich in blood supply, which help with any bone healing as well as decreasing bacterial inoculation.[25] Free flaps can be applied 3 to 5 days after initial debridement of necrotic bone and soft tissue.

One type of flap is the reverse sural artery flap.[25] The patient is placed in a prone position. The pedicle, approximately 4 to 5 cm in width, consisting of dermis, subcutaneous tissue, deep fascia, small saphenous vein, sural nerve, and accompanying sural and peroneal perforating arteries is marked on the posterior aspect of the leg between the 2 heads of the gastrocnemius muscle. The skin of the pedicle is elevated as a full thickness graft. Veins and nerves are ligated at the proximal border, and the flap and pedicle are lifted distally to the pivot point approximately 5 cm proximal to the lateral malleolus where the distal perforators leave the peroneal artery. The flap is then rotated through a subcutaneous tunnel and placed over the defect. There is no need for microsurgical anastomosis for this procedure. The donor site is then closed primarily or a skin graft is applied.

The saphenous flap is another option for closure of the heel. The patient is placed in a supine position for this procedure. The flap is outlined along the medial aspect of the knee to the medial malleolus, with the pivot point proximal to the medial malleolus. This pedicle is different from the sural flap in that it contains the great saphenous vein and the saphenous nerve.

Flaps containing abductor hallucis and abductor digiti minimi muscles are viable options but are often not chosen because of the small size of these muscles. However, they are used if the other free flaps would create too large of a functional loss. The abductor hallucis muscle flap has a pedicle from the posterior tibial artery, whereas the extensor digitorum muscle flap feeds from the dorsalis pedis artery. Rectus abduminus and gracilis muscles free flaps are other options available to close the wound.

Yildirim and colleagues[28] treated 9 patients with neurocutaneous flaps and reported 8 patients returning to presurgical ambulation status without accommodative shoes. However, normal shoe wear may not be feasible in all patients later, secondary to increased width and deformity of the soft tissue coverage compared with a normal foot. Patients may report a "walking on jelly" sensation. A complication that occurs when performing this procedure is breakdown of the flap because of the difference in pressure on the new flap. Germann[29] reported that diabetes mellitus significantly impairs the success of flaps. Overall, necrosis of flaps varies from 5% to 25%. In patients with diabetes mellitus, the rate of necrosis increases to 32%.

If all of the procedures fail or there is no feasible option, a below-knee amputation should be considered. This amputation is considered a last resort.

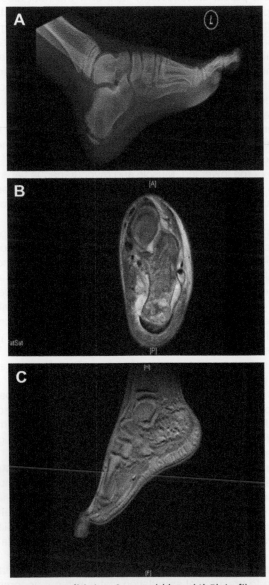

Fig. 5. Hematogenous osteomyelitis in a 9-year-old boy. (*A*) Plain film with patchy osteopenia about the calcaneus. (*B, C*) MRI revealing bone marrow edema of the calcaneus with abscess.

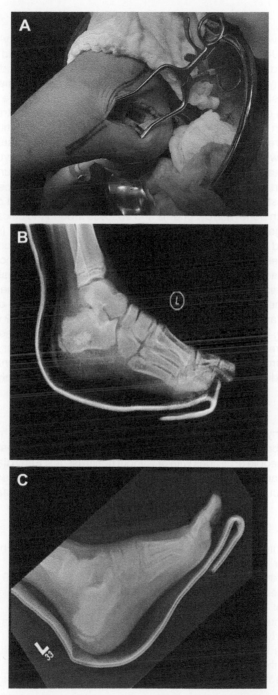

Fig. 6. (*A*) Intraoperative calcaneal window for placement of antibiotic beads for treatment of hematogenous osteomyelitis. (*B*) Immediate postoperative image. (*C*) 1-month postoperative image.

CASE STUDY

A 9-year-old boy was presented to the University Hospital, University of Medicine and Dentistry in New Jersey with persistent fever (temperature, 103°) and painful, edematous left ankle and foot for 2 weeks. No open lesions were noted and the patient was unable to bear any weight. The patient's mother stated that the patient had a pimple on the anterior distal tibia, which she popped before the onset of the pain. There was no recent trauma or travel outside of the country. The patient was treated at another hospital and given nafcillin with no relief of the pain or fever. Technetium Tc 99m bone scan showed increased uptake along the distal tibia. Laboratory results on admission were as follows: white blood cell count, 13,900 cells/mm³; erythrocyte sedimentation rate, 145 mm/h; and C-reactive protein level, 192 mg/dL. Blood cultures were positive for methicillin-sensitive *S aureus*. Radiographs revealed patchy osteopenia in the calcaneus suggestive of osteomyelitis (**Fig. 5**A). MRI demonstrated osteonecrosis of the calcaneus with bone marrow edema and abscess around the calcaneus. The diagnosis of hematogenous calcaneal osteomyelitis was then rendered (see **Fig. 5**B, C).

The patient had 2 incision and drainage procedures during the hospital admission. At the initial surgery, a lateral calcaneal window was made and vancomycin-absorbable antibiotic beads were inserted. Intraoperative cultures were consistent with methicillin-sensitive *S aureus*. The incision was closed primarily during the second incision and drainage. The patient received a peripherally inserted central catheter line and was on cefazolin and clindamycin for 4 weeks and then for another 2 weeks on amoxicillin/clavulanate. The patient remained non–weight bearing for 6 weeks. At the end of the 6 weeks of treatment, laboratory results revealed the following: white blood cell count, 5.8; erythrocyte sedimentation rate, 11; and C-reactive protein, 2 (**Fig. 6**). The patient was discharged after 3 months and was ambulating without any pain.

SUMMARY

Calcaneal osteomyelitis is seen more often in patients with neuropathy because of the increased risk of pressure ulcerations that can harbor pathogenic organisms. However, it can be seen in people of all ages with or without health issues. Early diagnosis is the key to successfully managing calcaneal osteomyelitis. Once an infection is realized, aggressive treatment should be started to prevent chronic osteomyelitis or drastic amputations.

REFERENCES

1. Nade S. Acute hematogenous osteomyelitis in infancy and childhood. J Bone Joint Surg Br 1983;65(2):109–19.
2. Lew DP, Waldvogel FA. Osteomyelitis. Lancet 2004;364:369–79.
3. Nixon GW. Hematogenous osteomyelitis of metaphyseal-equivalent locations. Am J Roentgenol 1978;130:123–9.
4. Trueta J. Three types of acute hematogenous osteomyelitis: a clinical and vascular study. J Bone Joint Surg Br 1959;41:671–80.
5. Cierny G, Mader JT, Penninck A. A clinical staging system for adult osteomyelitis. Contemp Orthop 1985;10:17–37.
6. Kelly PJ. Infected nonunion of the femur and tibia. Orthop Clin North Am 1984;15:481–90.
7. Cetinus E, Ciragil P, Uzel M, et al. Calcaneal osteomyelitis after puncture wound to foot: case report and review of the literature. J Orthopaed Traumatol 2005;6:194–6.
8. Ericson C, Lingren L, Lindbery L. Cloxacillin in the prophylaxis of post-operative infections of the hip. J Bone Joint Surg Am 1973;55:808–13.

9. Lee MC, Tashjian RZ, Eberson CP. Calcaneus osteomyelitis from community-acquired MRSA. Foot Ankle Int 2007;28(2):276–80.
10. Laughlin RT, Mader JT, Calhoun JH. Calcaneal osteomyelitis: an analysis of aetiology and pathogenic organisms. Foot Ankle Surg 1999;5:171–7.
11. Jaakkola J, Kehl D. Hematogenous calcaneal osteomyelitis in children. J Pediatr Orthop 1999;19:699–704.
12. Armstrong D, Lavery LA, Sariaya M, et al. Leukocytosis is a poor indicator of acute osteomyelitis of the foot in diabetes mellitus. J Foot Ankle Surg 1996;35:280–3.
13. Kaleta JL, Fleischli JW, Reilly CH. The diagnosis of osteomyelitis in diabetes using erythrocyte sedimentation rate: a pilot study. J Am Podiatr Med Assoc 2001; 91(9):445–50.
14. Grayson ML, Gibbons GW, Balogh K, et al. Probing to bone in infected pedal ulcers. A clinical sign of underlying osteomyelitis in diabetic patients. J Am Med Assoc 1995;273:721–3.
15. Lavery LA, Armstrong DG, Peters EJ, et al. Probe to bone test for foot osteomyelitis reliable or relic? Diabetes Care 2007;30(2):270–4.
16. Mackowiak PA, Jone SR, Smith JW. Diagnostic value of sinus tract cultures in chronic osteomyelitis. J Am Med Assoc 1978;239(26):2772–5.
17. Lavery LA, Sariaya M, Ashry H, et al. Microbiology of osteomyelitis in diabetic foot infections. J Foot Ankle Surg 1995;34:61–4.
18. Lipman BT, Collier BD, Carrera GF, et al. Detection of osteomyelitis in the neuropathic foot: nuclear medicine, MRI, and conventional radiography. Clin Nucl Med 1998;23(2):77–82.
19. Gold RH, Tong DJ, Crim JR, et al. Imaging the diabetic foot. Skeletal Radiol 1995; 24:563–71.
20. Schauwecker DS, Park HM, Mock BH, et al. Evaluation of complicating osteomyelitis with Tc-99m MDP, In-11 granulocytes and Ga-67 citrate. J Nucl Med 1984; 25(8):849–53.
21. Johnson JE, Kennedy EJ, Shereff MJ, et al. Prospective study of bone, Indium-111-labeled white blood cell, and gallium scanning for the evaluation of osteomyelitis in the diabetic foot. Foot Ankle Int 1996;17(1):10–6.
22. Chandnani VP, Beltran J, Morris CS, et al. Acute experimental osteomyelitis and abscesses: detection with MR imaging versus CT. Radiology 1990;174(1):233–6.
23. Mader JT, Mohan D, Calhoun J. A practical guide to the diagnosis and management of bone and joint infections. Drugs 1997;54:253–64.
24. Bollinger M, Thordarson D. Partial calcanectomy: an alternative to below knee amputation. Foot Ankle Int 2002;10:927–32.
25. Bragdon G, Baumhauer J. Total calcanectomy for the treatment of calcaneal osteomyelitis. Tech Foot Ankle Surg 2008;7(1):52–5.
26. Smith DG, Stuck RM, Ketner L, et al. Partial calcanectomy for the treatment of large ulcerations of the heel and calcaneal osteomyelitis. An amputation of the back of the foot. J Bone Joint Surg Am 1992;74:571–6.
27. Pontén B. The fasciocutaneous flap: its use in soft tissue defects of the lower leg. Br J Plast Surg 1981;34:215–20.
28. Yildirim S, Gideroglu K, Akoz T. The simple and effective choice for treatment of chronic calcaneal osteomyelitis: neurocutaneous flaps. Plast Reconstr Surg 2003; 111(2):753–60.
29. Germann G. Invited discussion: the simple and effective choice for treatment of chronic calcaneal osteomyelitis: neurocutaneous flaps. Plast Reconstr Surg 2003; 111:761–2.

Systemic Causes of Heel Pain

Eric Lui, DPM*

KEYWORDS

• Heel • Pain • Systemic • Plantar fasciitis

This article reviews the systemic causes of heel pain. Conditions discussed include rheumatoid arthritis, seronegative arthritides, metastatic disease, gout, sarcoidosis, Paget disease of bone, inflammatory bowel disease, infectious diseases, sickle cell anemia, and hyperparathyroidism. Diagnosis and treatment of the specific conditions are discussed to provide the podiatric physician with the clinical knowledge needed for proper treatment of patients with these conditions.

The treatment of heel pain can be a frustrating clinical course. Ninety percent of heel pain improves with conservative care, but the duration of the conservative care can vary.[1] There are cases that improve within the first several days or weeks of conservative treatment, whereas others may take 6 months or longer before improvement is seen. There is no defined period of time in which a person's heel pain will resolve. This unpredictability is because there are so many possible causes of heel pain: stress fracture, calcaneal apophysitis, bursitis, infection, bone tumor, plantar fasciitis, infracalcaneal bursitis, retained foreign body, neurogenic heel pain, insertional Achilles tendonitis, plantar fibroma, and systemic causes. However, there is a treatment of these causes of heel pain once the appropriate diagnosis is made.

The initial workup is familiar: the authors order radiographs to evaluate for the presence of a stress fracture, bone tumor, retained foreign body, or heel spur. The radiographs are usually negative for any osseous pathology. A plantar heel spur may be present but in most cases its presence is not the cause of the patient's pain (**Fig. 1**).

The patient should also be evaluated for the presence of a neurogenic cause such as a double crush or a tarsal tunnel syndrome. The patient is diagnosed with plantar fasciitis and usually instructed to use ice, rest, use over-the-counter orthoses, purchase new shoes, and perform stretching exercises. The patient is placed on a course of NSAIDs or a corticosteroid injection is administered. A strapping may be also applied to the affected foot. After 2 to 4 weeks, the patient returns, and usually the patient's heel pain has improved significantly. A few of those patients do not improve, and some may get worse. At this point neurogenic heel pain or a systemic

Connecticut Surgical Group, 85 Seymour Street #409, Hartford, CT 06106, USA
* 79-60 78th Avenue, Glendale, NY 11385.
E-mail address: ESOOGYLLIS@COMCAST.NET

Clin Podiatr Med Surg 27 (2010) 431–441
doi:10.1016/j.cpm.2010.04.004   podiatric.theclinics.com

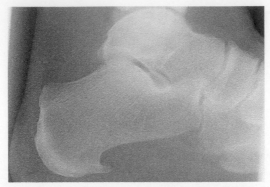

Fig. 1. Is the plantar heel spur here caused by a systemic process or is the cause strictly mechanical?

cause should be considered. Any radiographic changes not consistent with plantar fasciitis may indicate a systemic cause.

There are many systemic causes of heel pain, including rheumatoid arthritis, ankylosing spondylitis, psoriatic arthritis, inflammatory bowel disease, sarcoidosis, hyperparathyroidism, hematogenous osteomyelitis, metastatic disease, Paget disease, and sickle cell anemia. Sorting through all these systemic causes begins with a history and physical examination. A family history of a certain systemic disease can guide the physician toward a systemic cause for the patient's heel pain. This systemic cause can then be further evaluated with the appropriate testing.

The initial workup for a systemic cause of heel pain starts with a basic arthritic panel. This will consist of rheumatoid factor (RF), human leukocyte antigen 27 (HLA-B27), antinuclear antigen (ANA), and erythrocyte sedimentation rate (ESR)/c-reactive protein (CRP). RF can be positive in 75% to 85% of rheumatoid patients. HLA-B27 has a sensitivity of approximately 90% to 95% in ankylosing spondylitis, 80% in Reiter syndrome, 50% in inflammatory bowel disease, and 70% in psoriasis. ANA is positive in 95% of patients with systemic lupus erythematosus (SLE), but it can be seen in patients with rheumatoid arthritis and Sjogren disease. ESR/CRP are nonspecific and can be used to monitor the progression of an inflammatory process.[2,3]

RHEUMATOID ARTHRITIS

The onset of rheumatoid arthritis is between the third and fifth decade of life. The prevalence is approximately 0.8% in the world population with women affected 2 to 2.5 times more than men. RF is present in about 75% to 85% of patients with rheumatoid arthritis but can be increased in chronic bacterial infections and viral infections, parasitic diseases, and chronic inflammatory diseases. A positive RF has a sensitivity of approximately 66% and specificity of 83%. Anticyclic citrullinated peptide antibody (anti-CCP antibody) is normally positive with a sensitivity of 70% and a specificity of 95%. Anti-CCP and RF can present 10 years before the onset of symptoms and can be useful in starting preventative treatment. There seems to be a connection between the environment and genetic factors in the development of rheumatoid arthritis. There is an association of rheumatoid arthritis and human lymphocyte antigen DR1 or DR4. Eighty percent of Caucasians with rheumatoid arthritis express either subtype. There is a greater than 30% concordance rate between monozygotic twins.[3–6]

Diagnosis based on criteria set by the American College of Rheumatology[7]

1. Morning stiffness greater than 1 hour
2. Arthritis of 3 or more joint areas; right or left proximal interphalangeal joint (PIPJ), metacarpophalangeal joint (MCPJ), wrist, elbow, knee, ankle, and metatarsal phalangeal joint (MPJ)
3. Arthritis of hand joints (swelling in at least 1 area: wrist, PIPJ, or MCPJ)
4. Symmetric arthritis
5. Rheumatoid nodules
6. Serum RF
7. Radiographic changes.

The first 4 criteria must have been present for at least 6 weeks. Four out of 7 criteria must be present for the diagnosis of rheumatoid arthritis. Patients with 2 criteria are not excluded. This revised criterion has a sensitivity of 91% to 94% and a specificity of 89%.[7]

The inciting event in the development of rheumatoid arthritis is still unknown. It is hypothesized that a viral or bacterial infection may be the trigger to this inflammatory process. The primary pathologic findings in rheumatoid arthritis are synovial changes. There is damage to the endothelial lining of the microvasculature of the synovium resulting in proliferation of the superficial cell lining with edema and fibrin exudation. T lymphocytes invade the area and are followed later in the process by plasma cells. Neovascularization occurs, along with proliferation of the synovium forming pannus, which invades and erodes cartilage and bone. The physician should be attentive for complaints involving major joints such as the cervical spine, shoulders, elbows, hands/wrists, hips, knees, and the foot/ankle. Joint deformities to the hands and feet are characteristic and can be easily noted. However, attention should be paid to extra-articular manifestations and patient complaints such as the presence of rheumatoid nodules and vasculitic lesions, episcleritis, scleritis keratoconjunctivitis sicca, inflammation of the cricoarytenoid joint, pleurisy, pericardial manifestations, and hypochromic microcytic anemia.[3–5]

Radiographic findings particular to the calcaneus in rheumatoid arthritis include erosion of the bone along the posterior superior surface and the posterior surface above the insertion of the Achilles tendon. Retrocalcaneal and plantar spurs are also commonly seen.[8] The reason for development of plantar heel pain in rheumatoid arthritis is largely unknown. A study by Falsetti and colleagues[9] in 2004 revealed the presence of a pattern of inflammation and edema of the heel pad in 6.6% of patients with rheumatoid arthritis. Their ultrasound based study revealed the possibility that there is focal rupture of the fibrous septae of the heel pad along with necrosis of the fat pad. Most of the patients with this observed pattern had associated heel pain.

Treatment of rheumatoid arthritis centers on early diagnosis. The more the disease has progressed, the worse the prognosis. Once the disease is diagnosed, treatment needs to be aggressive to prevent joint destruction. The patient should be referred to a rheumatologist. Nonsteroidal antiinflammatory drugs (NSAIDs), disease-modifying antirheumatic drugs (DMARDs) and corticosteroids are used depending on the severity of the disease. Physical and occupational therapy should be instituted to retain joint function.

ANKYLOSING SPONDYLITIS

Ankylosing spondylitis mainly affects the spine and sacroiliac joint. Sacroiliitis is the first recognized clinical manifestation of the disease. The onset is in late adolescent or early adulthood and it is rarely seen to develop after the age of 40 years. Men are twice as likely to develop the disease as women. Its worldwide prevalence can range from 0.1% to 6%.

The disease initially presents as back pain in the gluteus or sacroiliac joint region. Clinical features of ankylosing spondilitis include sacroiliitis, spondylitis, arthritis of the hips and shoulders, peripheral arthritis, enthesitis, osteoporosis, spinal fracture, spondylodiscitis, pseudoarthrosis, acute anterior uveitis, and aortitis. The primary clinical feature is loss of spinal mobility, which can be evaluated through a Wright-Schober test.[3,10,11] The level of the fifth lumbar spinous is identified. Points 5 cm above and 10 cm below this level are then marked. The patient is then asked to bend over and touch his/her toes. The distance between the 2 points should increase in proportion to the spinal flexion range of motion.

The clinical diagnosis of ankylosing spondylitis is made based on the 1984 modified New York Criteria.

Radiologic criterion
    Sacroiliitis grade greater than or equal to 2 bilaterally, or
    Sacroiliitis grade 3 to 4 unilaterally (grade 1, - some loss of joint margins; grade 2, some sclerosis with erosion; grade 3, severe erosion of the joint with joint widening, ankylosis may or may not be present; grade 4, complete ankylosis)
Clinical criteria
    Low-back pain and stiffness greater than 3 months that improves with exercise but not rest
    Limitation of motion of the lumbar spine in the sagittal and frontal planes
    Limitation of chest expansion compared with normal values for age and sex.

The condition is definitely ankylosing spondylitis if the radiologic criterion is associated with at least 1 clinical criterion.[12]

Enthesitis of ankylosing spondilitis, which is inflammation of the attachment points of ligaments and capsule (enthesis),[13] can lead to insertional Achilles tendonitis and plantar fasciitis. Posterior and plantar heel pain can present clinically, differentiating ankylosing spondylitis from typical heel pain. The insertional Achilles tendonitis is commonly accompanied by an effusion of the retrocalcaneal bursa. Radiographs can reveal the presence of a fluffy periosteal reaction at this site. In addition, the following radiographic findings may be seen: erosion of the posterior aspect of the calcaneus superior to the Achilles tendon insertion, retrocalcaneal spur at the site of insertion of the Achilles tendon, and erosion of the plantar aspect of the calcaneus distal to the origin of the plantar fascia.[8]

However, the most common radiographic findings are seen in the sacroiliac joint. Osteitis and osseous erosion are features of the disease at points of ligamentous or tendonous attachment. Infiltration with plasma cells, macrophages, mast cells, lymphocytes, and chondrocytes results in erosion and sclerosis. Continuation of the disease process leads to replacement of local tissues with fibrocartilage that will eventually ossify. This process is seen with the development of a bamboo spine, pathognomonic for ankylosing spondylitis.[2,3,11,13]

HLA-B27 is seen in more than 90% of patients with ankylosing spondylitis and has a sensitivity of approximately 95%. Increased CRP and ESR are seen in 50% to 75% of patients with ankylosing spondylitis. Increased immunoglobulin A (IgA) is also noted in these patients. Fifteen percent of patients have a mild normocytic, normochromic anemia.

Ankylosing spondylitis predominately affects the ankle and heel rather than the forefoot. The lack of dermatologic features distinguishes this disease from other seronegative arthropathies. Treatment of ankylosing spondylitis consists of early diagnosis, NSAIDs, and daily exercises.[2,3,11,13] Heel pain is treated with the usual modalities.

PSORIATIC ARTHRITIS

Psoriatic arthritis has had a reported prevalence of approximately 0.3% to 1%. Psoriasis is seen between the ages of 5 and 15 years, with the onset of psoriatic arthritis between the ages of 30 and 55 years. The distribution between men and women is fairly equal. The clinical presentation is divided into 3 groups: asymmetric oligoarthritis or monoarthritis, polyarthritis, or axial disease. The calcaneus and forefoot are more commonly affected than the remainder of pedal joints or ankle in psoriatic arthritis.[14] Often the presenting heel pain will be unilateral. Dermatologic presentations include silvery scaled, erythematous plaques along extensor surfaces and nail changes including pitting, and brown-yellow discoloration, also known as the oil drop sign. Nail changes are predictive of those patients who will develop psoriatic arthritis.[2,3,11]

The Auspitz sign is the presence of pin-point bleeding after lifting of the scales. Radiographic features unique to psoriatic arthritis are a combination of osseous erosions with new bone production. The following radiographic findings of the calcaneus can be noted in psoriatic arthritis: erosion of the posterior aspect of the calcaneus superior to the Achilles tendon insertion, retrocalcaneal spur at the site of insertion of the Achilles tendon, plantar heel spur at the origin of the plantar fascia, and erosion of the plantar aspect of the calcaneus distal to the origin of the plantar fascia.[8] Another finding in the foot is a pencil-in-cup deformity in which there is erosion and tapering of the proximal phalanx with osseous proliferation of the distal phalanx. The interphalangeal joint of the hallux is also commonly a site of destruction during the disease process.[11] Enthesitis is a common feature of the disease and can cause heel pain through inflammation of the insertion of the Achilles tendon and origin of the plantar fascia.[15] An effusion of the retrocalcaneal bursa is also often present. These features distinguish heel pain due to a seronegative arthritide from typical heel pain.

Treatment of the disease consists of topical agents for skin lesions, NSAIDs, disease DMARDs (methotrexate, sulfasalazine), tumor necrosis factor inhibitors, and photochemotherapy.[3,14] The heel pain can be treated with NSAIDs, injections, and physical therapy.

REITER SYNDROME

Reiter syndrome is a reactive syndrome consisting of nongonococcal urethritis, arthritis, and conjunctivitis. The disease predominantly affects men and can present between the ages of 13 and 60 years. *Chlamydia trachomatis* is the most common cause of urethritis and the reactive arthritis is triggered by this organism. Other causative organisms include *Campylobacter*, *Salmonella*, *Shigella*, and *Yersinia*.[2,3] Conjunctivitis is present concomitantly or lags behind the presenting symptoms of urethritis.

The lower extremities are more commonly affected than the upper extremities. Inflammatory arthritis of the hindfoot is highly characteristic of Reiter disease. When the digits are involved, there is sausage-type swelling.[2,3,13] Enthesitis is a common finding, as with other seronegative arthritides, and leads to plantar and posterior heel pain along with an effusion of the retrocalcaneal bursa, differentiating it from typical heel pain. Sixty-one percent of patients with Reiter syndrome present with heel pain.[16] Extra-articular manifestations include keratoderma blennorrhagicum, circinate balanitis, and oral ulcerations. Laboratory evaluation can reveal a mild, normocytic, normochromic anemia, leukocytosis, or thrombocytosis. The ESR and CRP are increased as well as IgA. Synovial fluid evaluation usually reveals a white blood cell count of 5000 to 50,000/μL, poor viscosity, poor mucin clot test, and turbidity. Reiter cells, which are large mononuclear cells with ingested polymorphonuclear leukocytes with inclusion bodies, may be present.[2,3]

Radiographic features of the disease include fluffy periosteal reaction at insertions of ligaments and tendons. This reaction can be seen at the insertion of the Achilles tendon and origin of the plantar fascia. Erosion of the superior and posterior aspect of the calcaneus can be seen. An irregular plantar heel spur due to erosion and bone formation at the origin of the plantar fascia will commonly be noted.[8] Spontaneous fusion of the hindfoot or midfoot in a young man indicates chronic Reiter syndrome.

The presence of nongonococcal urethritis or cervicitis and peripheral arthritis has been defined by the American College of Rheumatology as preliminary criteria for Reiter syndrome.[2] However, the diagnosis of Reiter syndrome is primarily based on clinical and laboratory findings. Patients in whom Reiter syndrome is suspected should be carefully examined for the extra-articular manifestations described earlier. Reiter syndrome is a self-limiting disease that usually resolves within a year. However, some patients will continue to have chronic musculoskeletal problems. Chronic foot pain specifically in the joints of the hindfoot and heel pain are the major clinical symptoms.[2,11,13]

Treatment of Reiter disease mainly involves the use of NSAIDs, local injections, and physical therapy. Maintaining motion of the affected joints is important to prevent fusion. The usefulness of antibiotics in the disease process is not known.

The use of ciprofloxacin, doxycycline, and erythromycin has shown mixed results.[3]

INFLAMMATORY BOWEL DISEASE

Inflammatory bowel disease, consisting of Crohn disease and ulcerative colitis, results in arthritis in 10% to 20% of patients affected. The arthritis is of a migratory nature and tends to affect the joints of the lower extremities. Pyoderma gangrenosa is seen with ulcerative colitis and erythema nodosum is seen with Crohn disease.[2,3] The cause is unknown but it is believed to be due to an altered relationship between the immune system and commensal microflora and intestinal antigens.[17] The disease tends to affect young adults or children. The ankle joint is affected in 38% of patients with Crohn disease.[11] Common laboratory features include a positive perinuclear antineutrophil cytoplasmic antibody (pANCA; present in 60% of patients with ulcerative colitis), leukocytosis, and increased ESR/CRP.

The arthritic process is not destructive and usually subsides with treatment of the inflammatory bowel disease. Colectomy in ulcerative colitis usually results in resolution of the arthritis process. Colectomy in Crohn disease does not yield the same results. Sulfasalazine, tumor necrosis factor inhibitors, and NSAIDs are the standards in treatment of the arthritic process. NSAIDs should be used with caution in inflammatory bowel disease.[2,3] Local injections can also be used.

SARCOIDOSIS

Sarcoidosis is more prevalent in the African American population than in the White population. The disease process presents between 20 and 40 years of age. It is a granulomatous disease that can affect all organ systems and can produce rheumatic manifestations in 10% to 15% of patients. There are 2 forms of arthritis that can manifest in this disease; an early form and a later form. The early form presents within 6 months of the presentation of sarcoidosis. It will generally involve the ankles with possible spread to involve the knees, wrists, elbows, PIPJs, and metacarpalphalangeal joints. The arthritis presents as polyarthritis that is symmetric and additive. Erythema nodosum is seen in 66% of the cases of early arthritis. Lofgren syndrome is a clinical variant of sarcoidosis consisting of arthritis, bilateral hilar adenopathy, and erythema nodosum. This form of arthritis has a good prognosis and usually resolves within 3 months.[2,3,6] Heel pain can be a common finding in the early stage. Shaw and colleagues[18] reported that all of the patients in their study had heel pain during the acute stage of the disease, albeit with a sample size of only 7.

The second form of arthritis presents 6 months or later after the initial presentation of sarcoidosis. This form of arthritis is significantly less severe than the early form. The most common site of involvement is the knees. There is involvement of the ankles and PIPJs. Clinical signs include cutaneous sarcoidosis and dactylitis. Cutaneous sarcoidosis can consist of papules, plaques, and nodules. Violaceous facial plaques (lupus pernio) are associated with chronic sarcoidosis. There is an absence of erythema nodosum in this form. Radiographic features include punched out cystic type lesions in osseous sarcoid.[2,3,6]

Sarcoidosis can present as bilateral heel pain. Diagnosis of sarcoidosis is based on the clinical presentation along with the histological findings. When cutaneous lesions are present a transbronchial lung biopsy can be positive in 90% of patients with sarcoidosis. A Kveim-Siltzbach test can also be performed. A suspension of spleen or lymph node containing granulomas is injected intradermally. A positive test produces a granulomatous inflammatory reaction with papule formation.[2] Treatment options included NSAIDs, glucocorticoids, steroid-sparing agents (ie, methotrexate, imuran, plaquenil), injection therapy, tumor necrosis factor inhibitors, and antimalarial drugs.

PAGET DISEASE OF BONE

Paget disease of bone is a benign neoplastic process that affects the formation of bone. There is alteration of bone resorption with destruction. The resultant repair process results in an irregular mosaic pattern. This pattern is due to the presence of mature and immature bone structure. Radiographs may reveal areas of increased density along with areas of lucency. Patchiness is often described as a result of the turnover of bone in these areas (**Fig. 2**).

The most commonly affected sites are the skull, tibia, pelvis, femur, and vertebral bodies. Involvement of the heel has been reported in the literature. A study by Claustre and colleagues[19] involved 100 patients, 20 of whom had involvement of the calcaneus. However, only 2 of the 20 patients reported the presence of heel pain. A case report by Perrot and colleagues[20] presented 2 patients with Paget disease with intractable heel pain as the presenting symptom.

Diagnosis of Paget disease of bone is based on an increase of serum alkaline phosphatase and on radiograph findings. The anatomic regions involved can be evaluated with a 3-phase bone scan. Treatment of the underlying Paget disease with bisphosphonate therapy will usually resolve the heel pain. NSAIDs can be used as adjunctive therapy for treatment of pain and inflammation.[2]

INFECTIOUS CAUSES OF HEEL PAIN

One cause of heel pain that can be overlooked is an infection. Hematogenous osteomyelitis of the calcaneus has been reported in between 1.5% and 10% of all cases of

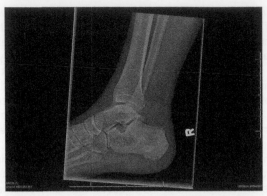

Fig. 2. A 55-year-old man who presented with posterior heel pain. There is trabecular coarsening along with cortical thickening of the calcaneus. There are also areas of increased osseous density. Paget disease of the calcaneus is evident here.

hematogenous osteomyelitis in children. A presentation of heel pain in a child is normally diagnosed as calcaneal apophysitis, which is easily treated with ice and a stretching regimen. Recalcitrant heel pain in a child should raise the possibility of hematogenous osteomyelitis. Possible causative agents include *Staphylococcus aureus*, *Staphylococcus epidermidis*, group B and D *Streptococcus*, with *S aureus* being the most common. Tuberculous osteomyelitis is another consideration in heel pain. The causative agent is *Mycobacterium tuberculosis*. A 16 to 19 month period of time between initial presentation and diagnosis of osteomyelitis due to tuberculosis has been reported in studies. A purified protein derivative and chest radiograph can be negative despite the presence of tuberculous osteomyelitis.[16] For a more detailed discussion, see the section on calcaneal osteomyelitis.

METASTATIC DISEASE

Between 20% and 30% of patients with malignancy will have metastases to osseous structures. Metastases to the hand account for 0.007% to 0.3% of metastatic disease to osseous structures.[21] Metastatic disease to the foot is about one-half to one-third of the rates seen in the hand. In a review of 694 patients with metastatic disease by Maheshwari and colleagues,[21] there were 14 cases of metastases to the foot. The calcaneus was involved in 6 of those cases, which correlate with the calcaneus as the most common site of metastases to the foot. The genitourinary system was the most common site of primary disease. In the literature, other common sites of primary disease with osseous metastases have been found to include the lung, the kidneys, the breast, and the colorectal system. It has been theorized that supradiaphragmatic disease tends to metastasize to the hands and subdiaphragmatic disease tends to metastasize to the feet.[22–24]

Presentation of the metastatic disease of the foot has been noted up to 172 months after diagnosis of the primary neoplasm. The average time to diagnosis of metastatic disease of the foot has been reported to be up to 24 months after initial presentation of the disease.[25] This may be to the result of confusion with other disease processes and inappropriate treatment. The clinical evidence can mimic fracture, arthritides, crystalline deposition disease, infection, and other disorders that result in a red, hot, swollen, and painful foot. Radiographs may reveal the presence of lytic or blastic osseous lesions. Correct diagnosis can be obtained through a biopsy of the lesion. The survival rate of patients with metastatic disease to the foot is low given the delay in presentation and diagnosis. Once metastatic disease is diagnosed, consultation and treatment in conjunction with a surgical oncologist is essential.[23]

HYPERPARATHYROIDISM

Hyperparathyroidism is a metabolic disorder in which parathyroid hormone is secreted in excess. This overproduction of the hormone results in osteoporosis. Clinical signs of hyperparathyroidism include hypercalcemia, recurrent kidney stones, mental status changes, fatigue, depression, gastrointestinal distress, and back pain. Fishco and colleagues[26] presented a case of recalcitrant heel pain initially diagnosed as plantar fasciitis. On presentation, the patient had a medical history significant for multiple spinal fractures, recurrent kidney stones, and gastrointestinal disease. The patient was later diagnosed with a stress fracture of the calcaneus secondary to hyperparathyroidism. The patient's serum calcium was normal but her parathyroid hormone was greatly increased. An iliac crest bone biopsy confirmed the diagnosis.

GOUT

Crystalline deposition disease such as gout usually presents clinically in joints. This disease process is due to the overproduction or undersecretion of uric acid. Uric acid crystals are negative birefringent and are needle shaped. The first MPJ of the foot is the most commonly affected site in the foot. Radiographically, osseous erosions, described as rat-bite lesions, of the first metatarsal head are commonly seen. Heel pain can manifest secondary to the presence of tophaceous deposits about the calcaneus, specifically about the Achilles tendon and its insertion. For symptomatic tophaceous deposits, surgical excision may be indicated.[6]

SICKLE CELL ANEMIA

Sickle cell anemia causes thromboses of the microvascular circulation supplying bones, which results in aseptic necrosis. Aseptic necrosis of the calcaneus has been reported in the literature, but is rare.[6] Radiographic findings include patchy sclerosis, cortical thickening, and osteopenia.

Allen and Andrews[27] presented a case of an African American man with sickle cell anemia who developed severe bilateral heel pain. A bone scan revealed decreased uptake in the calcanei, which is consistent with aseptic necrosis. Rothschild and Sebes[28] conducted a study that evaluated 100 patients with sickle cell anemia. They discovered erosions of the posterior superior aspect of the calcaneus in 14% of their patients and believed this to be pathognomonic for sickle cell anemia. Allen and Andrews[27] questioned this finding and believed that aseptic necrosis may have played a role in the observations. Milner and Burke[29] reported a case of aseptic necrosis of the calcaneus in a patient with sickle cell anemia. Lally and colleagues[30] presented a case with aseptic necrosis of the calcaneus in a patient with sickle cell trait. Aseptic necrosis in sickle cell trait is a rare finding, as it is in sickle cell anemia.

SUMMARY

The clinical course of heel pain can be frustrating to the clinician and the patient. Most heel pain responds to conservative care in a short period of time. However, other causes should be considered, especially if the heel pain is recalcitrant to treatment. A detailed history and physical examination, along with appropriate laboratory tests and radiological studies, can direct the physician toward the correct diagnosis. There are many systemic causes of heel pain, some common and others uncommon. Regardless of the incidence, a strong index of suspicion is raised whenever the heel pain fails to respond as routine plantar fasciitis should.

REFERENCES

1. Toomey EP. Plantar heel pain. Foot Ankle Clin 2009;14:229–45.
2. Klippel JH. Primer on the rheumatic diseases. Atlanta (GA): Arthritis Foundation; 1997.
3. Klippel JH, Stone JH, Crofford LJ, et al. Primer on the rheumatic diseases. 13th edition. New York: Arthritis Foundation; 2008.
4. Rindfleisch JA, Muller D. Diagnosis and management of rheumatoid arthritis. Am Fam Physician 2005;72:1037–47.
5. Jaakkola JI, Mann RA. A review of rheumatoid arthritis affecting the foot and ankle. Foot Ankle Int 2004;25:866–74.
6. Lichniak JE. The heel in systemic disease. Clin Podiatr Med Surg 1990;7:225–41.
7. Arnett FC, Edworthy SM, Bloch DA, et al. The American Rheumatism Association 1987 revised criteria for the classification of rheumatoid arthritis. Arthritis Rheum 1988;31:315–24.
8. Resnick D, Feingold MS, Curd J, et al. Calcaneal abnormalities in articular disorders, rheumatoid arthritis, ankylosing spondylitis, psoriatic arthritis and Reiter's syndrome. Radiology 1977;125:355–66.
9. Falsetti P, Frediani B, Acciai C, et al. Heel fat pad involvement in rheumatoid arthritis and in spondyloarthropathies: an ultrasonographic study. Scand J Rheumatol 2004;33:327–31.
10. Sieper J, Braun J, Rudwaleit M, et al. Ankylosing spondylitis: an overview. Ann Rheum Dis 2002;61:iii8–18.
11. Moll JM. Seronegative arthropathies in the foot. Seronegative arthropathies in the foot. Baillieres Clin Rheumatol 1987;1:289–315.
12. Van der Linden S, Valkenburg HA, Cats A. Evaluation of diagnostic criteria for ankylosing spondylitis. A proposal for modification of the New York criteria. Arthritis Rheum 1984;27:361–8.
13. Bluestone R. Collagen diseases affecting the foot. Foot Ankle 1982;2:311–7.
14. Bezza A, Niamane R, Amine B, et al. Involvement of the foot in patients with psoriatic arthritis: a review. Joint Bone Spine 2004;71:546–9.
15. Lehman TJ. Enthesitis, arthritis and heel pain. J Am Podiatr Med Assoc 1999;89: 18–9.
16. Kosinski M, Lilja E. Infectious causes of heel pain. J Am Podiatr Med Assoc 1999; 89:20–3.
17. Baumgart DC. What's new in inflammatory bowel disease in 2008? World J Gastroenterol 2008;14:329–30.
18. Shaw RA, Holt A, Stevens MB. Heel pain in sarcoidosis. Ann Intern Med 1988; 109:675–7.
19. Claustre J, Blotman F, Simon L. Heel involvement in Paget's disease of bone. Rev Rhum Mal Osteoartic 1976;43:43–5.
20. Perrot S, Mortier E, Renoux M, et al. Monostotic Paget's disease involving the calcaneus. Diagnostic and therapeutic problems. Two case-reports. Rev Rhum Engl Ed 1995;62:45–7.
21. Maheshwari AV, Chiappetta G, Kugler CD, et al. Metastatic skeletal disease of the foot: case reports and literature review. Foot Ankle Int 2008;29:699–710.

22. Libson E, Bloom RA, Husband JE, et al. Metastatic tumors of bones of the hand and foot. A comparative review and report of 43 additional cases. Skeletal Radiol 1987;16:387–92.
23. Groves MJ, Stiles RG. Metastatic breast cancer presenting as heel pain. J Am Podiatr Med Assoc 1998;88:400–5.
24. Berlin SJ, Mirkin GS, Tubridy SP. Tumors of the heel. Clin Podiatr Med Surg 1990; 7:307–21.
25. Hattrup SJ, Amadio PC, Sim FH, et al. Metastatic tumors of the foot and ankle. Foot Ankle 1998;8:243–7.
26. Fishco WD, Stiles RG. Atypical heel pain. Hyperparathyroidism induced stress fracture of the calcaneus. J Am Podiatr Med Assoc 1999;89:413–8.
27. Allen BJ, Andrews BS. Bilateral aseptic necrosis of calcanei in an adult male with sickle cell disease treated by a surgical coring procedure. J Rheumatol 1983;10: 294–6.
28. Rothschild BM, Sebes JI. Calcaneal abnormalities and erosive bone disease associated with sickle cell anemia. Am J Med 1981;71:427–30.
29. Milner P, Burke G. Isolated infarction of the os calcis in an adult. Clin Nucl Med 1993;18:530–1.
30. Lally EV, Buckley WM, Claster S. Diaphyseal bone infarctions in a patient with sickle cell trait. J Rheumatol 1983;10:813–6.

Painful Prominences of the Heel

Steven D. Vyce, DPM[a,b,c,*], Eliza Addis-Thomas, DPM[d],
Erin E. Mathews, DPM[d], Sonya L. Perez, DPM[d]

KEYWORDS

• Heel pain • Exostoses • Calcaneus • Peroneal trochlea

Heel pain is a common malady, with reported prevalence ranging from 4% to 21%.[1,2] Referral to foot and ankle specialists for heel pain is also common, but patient awareness of the cause of heel pain may be limited. Many misconceptions about how heel exostoses relate to heel pain exist in the medical community and the general patient population, with many patients referred for or presenting with the simple complaint "I have a heel spur." This article reviews the common exostoses of the heel, including plantar, lateral, and posterior spurs, with specific attention to the cause and treatments.

ANATOMY OF THE HEEL

The heel is the body's initial contact with the ground during normal gait. Each heel experiences loads up to 80% of body weight during heel strike of normal gait.[3] The calcaneus makes up most of the heel. It is roughly rectangular with multiple normal projections and prominences. The insertion of the Achilles tendon, origins of the intrinsic musculature of the foot, and numerous ligamentous attachments exert pull on various portions of the calcaneus, which cause normal prominences.

Medially, the shelf-like sustentaculum tali projects roughly parallel to the weight-bearing surface in the distal one-third of the bone. Laterally, the peroneal trochlea (or tubercle), a smaller retrotrochlear eminence, and the tubercle for the calcaneofibular ligament project from the otherwise smooth lateral wall. The anterior process of the calcaneus is normally small and rounded, projecting anterolaterally. The plantar tuberosity is the posteroplantar portion of the calcaneus and has a medial and a lateral

The authors wish to thank Gerald Gorecki, DPM, for his assistance in editing the manuscript.
[a] Department of Orthopaedics and Rehabilitation, Yale University School of Medicine, New Haven, CT, USA
[b] Yale/VACT PM&S-36, USA
[c] Podiatry Section, VA Connecticut Healthcare Systems, West Haven, CT, USA
[d] Yale-New Haven Hospital, 20 York Street, New Haven, CT, USA
* Corresponding author. VA Connecticut Healthcare Systems, Surgery Department, MS 112, 950 Campbell Avenue, West Haven, CT 06516.
E-mail address: Steven.Vyce@Yale.edu

Clin Podiatr Med Surg 27 (2010) 443–462
doi:10.1016/j.cpm.2010.04.005
0891-8422/10/$ – see front matter. Published by Elsevier Inc.

podiatric.theclinics.com

process. The anterior tubercle is a projection on the plantar surface distally, just behind the calcaneocuboid articulation. On the posterosuperior surface, the superior aspect of the posterior facet projects upwards; the posterosuperior aspect of the calcaneus may protrude slightly upwards and posteriorly and is called the bursal projection.[4] Although each of these structures Is expected anatomically, any one of them could become enlarged or hypertrophic.

LATERAL WALL

The peroneal trochlea or tubercle projects from the lateral wall below the posterior aspect of the posterior facet. The peroneal trochlea separates the peroneus brevis tendon above it and the peroneus longus tendon below it, and the peroneal retinaculum inserts at the tip of the tubercle. Grooves exist above and below the trochlea for the tendons, with variable depth.[4] Hyer and colleagues[5] reported a 90% prevalence of the tubercle but classified 43% of these as "flat."

An enlarged peroneal tubercle causing tenosynovitis of the peroneal tendons was first described by Burman,[6,7] and many case reports have been presented since then.[6–14] Enlargement or hypertrophy of the tubercle has been reported in up to 30% of tubercles.[7,8]

Symptoms associated with an enlarged peroneal tubercle may include localized pain to palpation, prominence, irritation or hyperkeratosis formation, bursitis, sural nerve entrapment, stiffness, pain with active range of motion (AROM)/passive range of motion (PROM) of the peroneals, and chronic lateral hindfoot pain.[6–14] Diagnosis can often be made by correlating radiographs to clinical symptoms. The enlarged tubercle is usually visualized on a calcaneal axial radiograph (**Fig. 1**). If symptomatic, magnet resonance imaging (MRI) should be considered

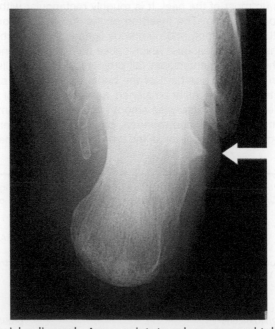

Fig. 1. Calcaneal axial radiograph. Arrow points to enlarge peroneal tubercle.

for further assessment of the integrity of the peroneal tendons, and the tubercle can be further assessed (**Figs. 2** and **3**). Attention should also be given to assess for the presence of an os peroneum, because the presence of an enlarged tubercle and os peroneum has been reported.[9]

Treatment consists of the typical conservative measures of rest, ice, physical therapy, and bracing followed by surgical excision for recalcitrant cases. Various techniques have been described, from simple excision or reduction in size of the tubercle[9] to lifting an osteochondral flap, removing underlying bone, and then replacing the flap to maintain smooth gliding of the peroneal tendons.[10] Tenosynovectomy and repair of the peroneal retinaculum are also usually performed. Although there are no large studies available, good results with return to normal function postoperatively can be expected. Ochoa and Banerjee[11] presented a case of recurrent symptoms 4 months after minimal incision-excision of the tubercle. A small recurrent tubercle was found concurrent with a longitudinal peroneus brevis tear. They performed a repeat tubercle resection, placed bone wax on the site, and repaired the tendon tear. The patient had complete resolution of symptoms.

ANTERIOR PROCESS

The anterior process of the calcaneus is located on the distal superior aspect of the calcaneus. The proximal dorsal surface of the anterior process is rough, with attachments for the extensor digitorum brevis and inferior extensor retinaculum. The anterior process may be enlarged, straightened or hook-like, and is almost always associated with a tarsal coalition in these instances.[4,15] This is referred to as the anteater sign. More information and treatment can be obtained in texts on tarsal coalition.

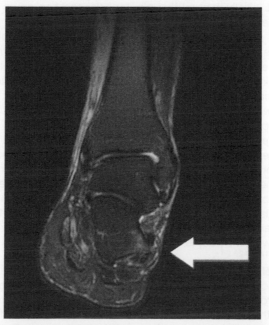

Fig. 2. Coronal MRI, T2 image. Arrow points to an enlarged peroneal tubercle that has increased signal intensity indicating edema of bone.

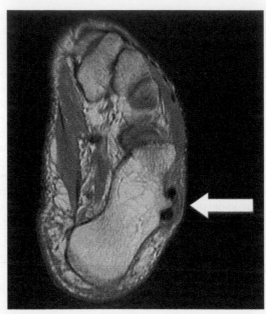

Fig. 3. Transverse MRI, T1 image. Arrow points to an enlarged peroneal tubercle, with peroneal tendons on either side of it.

PLANTAR HEEL

Plantar calcaneal osseous spurring was first described in 1900 by Plettner, a German physician.[16] It was initially thought that plantar calcaneal heel spurs were the primary cause of plantar heel pain. Current studies contradict this, however, and it is reported that 11% to 16% of the young to middle-aged population have plantar heel spurs without symptoms.[17–20] Although most plantar heel spurs are asymptomatic, there is a correlation between heel pain and plantar spurring. Shama and colleagues[19] reported a 13.2% incidence of heel spurs with only 31% of these patients being symptomatic. Approximately 75% of patients with heel pain have a spur.[19,21,22] Only one-third of patients with spurs show symptoms, whereas three-quarters of those with symptoms have spurs.

In a study of elderly patients aged between 62 and 94 years, Menz and colleagues[16] found that calcaneal spurs were present in 55% of the patients and were related to obesity, osteoarthritis, and current or previous heel pain. The strongest association was found with obesity; 45% of the patients with heel spurs were classified as obese, whereas only 9% of the nonobese participants had spurs. Patients with plantar calcaneal spurs were also more likely to have Achilles tendon spurs.[16] Other research has confirmed that plantar calcaneal spurs are more commonly found in older patients, obese patients, women, people with osteoarthritis, and people with previous or current heel pain.[17–20,23,24]

The classic heel spur is an osteophytic outgrowth projecting anteriorly from the plantar medial calcaneal tuberosity (**Fig. 4**). The outgrowth usually extends the entire width of the tuberosity or approximately 2.0 or 2.5 cm.[25–28] Also present in this area are the origins of the plantar fascia and intrinsic musculature of the foot. Some investigators believe that the plantar spur forms at the origin of the plantar fascia; others have suggested that spurs form at the origin of the intrinsic musculature. One study

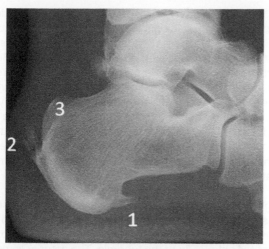

Fig. 4. Lateral radiograph of foot. 1, Typical plantar spur; 2, retrocalcaneal spur; 3, bursal projection of the calcaneus.

suggests that spurs originate in the flexor digitorium brevis muscle rather than inferiorly in the plantar fascia.[25] The same study also indicates that plantar spurs can form at the origins of the quadratus plantae, the long plantar ligament, the abductor hallucis muscle, and the abductor digitimi minimi muscle.

In a cadaveric study by Foreman and Green,[26] the plantar fascia was found to run under the calcaneus and remain plantar to the calcaneal spur. They found that the spur formation was at the origin of the flexor digitorium brevis and that the abductor hallucis can also contribute to the exostosis. Foreman and Green found in their cadaver specimen that the abductor digiti minimi and quadratus plantae muscle origins were lateral and superior to the spur, respectively (**Fig. 5**).

The cause of plantar heel spurs is not entirely clear. As previously stated, many investigators believe that the steady pulling of the plantar fascia causes an inflammatory process at the calcaneus. This constant pulling leads to periostitis that progresses

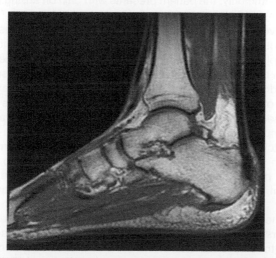

Fig. 5. Sagittal MRI, T1 image. Plantar spur above the level of the plantar fascia.

to osteogenesis.[29–31] This theory is called the longitudinal traction hypothesis.[31] Chang and Miltner[32] showed in histologic studies that there was chronic inflammation of the periosteum of calcaneal spurs with areas of fibrosis, necrosis, and sclerosis.

The vertical compression hypothesis proposed by Kumai and Benjamin[33] argues that spurring results from repetitive compressive forces rather than repetitive traction. They believe that calcaneal spurs are fibrocartilaginous outgrowths that form to protect the calcaneus from microcracks and stress fractures. A study by Li and Muehleman[34] found that the spur is generally not formed parallel to the plantar fascia or musculature. In addition, Li and Muehleman proposed that the spur develops in the direction of calcaneal stress during walking and standing. This theory is supported by other studies that suggest that plantar heel spurs are more common in overweight patients and in patients with decreased elasticity of the plantar fat pad, such as the elderly.[35,36]

Graham[17] thought that plantar heel exostoses were the result of the calcaneus healing itself, and the spur formed by the layering of calcification on top of the flexor digitorium muscle. In his study, technetium 99m scans were used to demonstrate increased uptake at the anterior lip of the tubercle. The anterior lip collapses because of the pull of the intrinsic muscles leading to the aforementioned healing process.[20]

In 1957, DuVries[28] described 3 types of calcaneal spurs. The first type of spur is large and asymptomatic; there is no pain associated with these spurs, because the spur is located on a non–weight-bearing surface. If there are associated inflammatory changes, they are usually subacute. It is usually an incidental finding on radiographic examination. DuVries also describes a large, painful spur that occurs when there is a depression of the weight-bearing arch. This alters the pitch of the calcaneus and the spur is in a weight-bearing location. These patients complain of pain with weight bearing from inflammation of the intrinsic musculature and bursa formation. The third type are spurs with minimal bony proliferation and irregular, uneven edges. These small spurs are usually found at the origin of the plantar fascia.[28]

HEEL SPUR SYNDROME

Heel spur syndrome is more accurately described as plantar fasciitis, which is a clinical diagnosis. Most commonly, the patient presents with pain on arising in the morning or after periods of rest; this has been called poststatic dyskinesia.[15] The pain typically improves with several steps but then worsens as the day progresses. Generally, clinical examination usually reveals pain in 1 of 2 areas. The most common clinical finding is pain along the plantar medial and inferior medial wall of the calcaneus.[15] More infrequently, pain can be found along the central band of the plantar fasciitis.

Heel spur syndrome is typically treated successfully with conservative methods. Fewer than 10% of patients require surgical intervention, regardless of the conservative treatment used.[37] The exceptions include patients with bilateral symptoms and patients with symptoms longer than 1 year.[15]

Rest, ice, stretching and physical therapy, nonsteroidal antiinflammatory medications, changes in shoe gear, and orthotics have all been found to resolve the pain associated with plantar fasciitis.[38] Local corticosteroid injections are a common nonsurgical treatment, with the injection directed into the area of maximal tenderness.[15]

Surgical treatment should be reserved for patients for whom conservative treatment fails. DuVries[28] first described the classic heel spur resection. He used a medial horizontal approach to remove the fascia from the medial tuberosity and resect the spur. However, branches of the medial calcaneal nerve may be severed by this approach causing varying degrees of anesthesia to the heel and arch. Modifications have been made to make the incision more plantar to avoid these complications.

Plantar fasciotomy has been found to be the preferred method for treating heel pain associated with plantar fasciitis. Studies comparing fascial release only versus release and spur resection have reported no major differences in outcomes.[39] There are multiple ways to perform the fasciotomy including open, percutaneous, and endoscopic.

The open fasciotomy provides good visualization and allows additional pathologic lesions to be addressed if needed.[39] The incision is located on the plantar medial arch. The incision is deepened through subcutaneous tissue until the plantar fascia is visualized. The fascial margins are then isolated and with the toes in extension, the medial fascial band is severed. Disadvantages of the procedure include prolonged recovery period, potential wound complications, and risk of nerve injury.

Lane and London[40] published a retrospective report on the percutaneous plantar transverse incision. In this paper, the investigators described a procedure, whereby under fluoroscopy, a 25-gauge needle was placed at the distal tip of the spur or tuberosity of the calcaneus. Then, a 5-mm transverse incision was made at the needle-entry position, and a #15 blade was used to sharply release the medial half of the plantar fascia under fluoroscopy. Postoperatively, the patient was partial weight bearing with crutches for 3 days and then returned to weight bearing as tolerated in athletic shoes. The percutaneous approach is advantageous because it requires minimal soft tissue resection, minimal operative time, and is a simple technique with a quick return to activity. Painful scar and nerve injury are potential complications.

Endoscopic plantar fasciotomy was first described by Barrett and Day in 1991 as a single-portal technique that was later modified to a 2-portal approach. Bazaz and Ferkel[41] later described the 2-portal approach. The first portal is a vertical incision distal medial to the posterior aspect of the medial malleolus. A tunnel is then created through soft tissue plantar to the plantar fascia and a trochar is passed through to the lateral aspect of the foot. The trochar is aligned parallel to the floor with the toes pointing up. A short, 30° (4 mm) arthroscope is passed through the lateral portal. A triangular knife creates an initial hole in the plantar fascia; then a hook knife is repeatedly passed to release the medial plantar fascia until the flexor digitorum brevis muscle belly is seen. Next, the arthroscope is placed medially and the triangular blade placed laterally to release the deep fascia of the abductor hallucis. The patient is allowed partial weight bearing as tolerated with full weight bearing once the portals have healed. The advantages of the endoscopic approach include minimal soft tissue trauma, faster recovery time, and earlier return to activity.[41] Lack of exposure to the nerve of the abductor digiti quinti and variable resection of the plantar fascia are disadvantages.

After any of these plantar fascial releases, it is important to place the patient in orthotics to help support the foot.[39,40] Some of the late-term complications associated with this procedure are calcaneocuboid pain, medial column strain, and pain in the ball of the foot.

POSTERIOR HEEL

Posterior heel pain is often directly correlated with calcaneal prominences, and differential diagnoses such as Achilles tendinitis and retrocalcaneal or Achilles bursitis may also be indirectly related to prominences. Haglund syndrome is a painful condition in which there is pain and a clinical prominence at the posterosuperior aspect of the calcaneus.[42–45] Pain is often produced from the pressure of the shoe counter on this area of the heel and can be initially relieved by removing the offending source of pressure. Continued irritation can lead to inflammation of the anatomical retrocalcaneal bursa, Achilles tendinitis above the level of the insertion, and formation and inflammation of an adventitial bursa superficial to the Achilles tendon.

In contrast, retrocalcaneal exostoses or excess bone formation behind the calcaneus often leads to insertional Achilles tendinitis and pain with direct pressure on the spur versus 40 (42.5% positive) asymptomatic heels.[46] Calcification or ossification behind the calcaneus, separate from the normal anatomy, is referred to as retrocalcaneal exostosis, Achilles calcification, or insertional calcific Achilles tendinitis, tendinosis, or tendonopathy. For simplicity, retrocalcaneal exostosis is used in this article.

ANATOMY

The posterior heel complex is a relatively tight space comprising the posterior calcaneus, the plantaris, and Achilles tendons and their insertions, fibro-fatty tissue,[4] an anatomical bursa, and it may contain an adventitial bursa. The inferior third of the posterior calcaneus is usually rounded and forms part of the weight-bearing area of the heel.[4] The Achilles tendon inserts on the middle third of the posterior calcaneus, and there may be a shelf-like projection or overhanging of bone at the superior aspect of the insertion.[4] The Achilles insertion also extends medially, laterally, and plantarly on the calcaneus, connecting with the plantar fascia plantarly[4,47] and should be considered to have a crescent-shaped insertion instead of a rectangular-shaped insertion.[48] The medial extension of the Achilles was measured to extend to a mean of 3.5 mm anterior to the most posterior portion of the tuberosity, whereas the lateral extension only extends 1 mm anteriorly.[48] The superior third of the posterior calcaneus is called the bursal projection (see **Fig. 4**), and its posterior surface is also known as the trigonum Achilleum. The space between the Achilles and trigonum Achilleum is known as the retrocalcaneal recess, and a portion is filled with fatty tissue and a bursa called the retrocalcaneal bursa[49] or deep retrocalcaneal bursa.[4] The retrocalcaneal recess is contiguous with the Kager triangle. Canoso and colleagues[50] identified via MRI, and Theobald and colleagues[51] later confirmed via ultrasound, MRI and anatomic dissection that a small tongue-like wedge of fat is present, and it shifts its position relative to the foot position. In plantar flexion, the wedge was seen to move into the retrocalcaneal recess between the Achilles and bursal projection. From neutral position to the dorsiflexed position, however, it was seen to move superior to the bursal projection, leaving the Achilles tendon in direct contact with the bursal projection. Canoso and colleagues[50] also showed that the wedge was prevented from moving into the recess in a patient with spondyloarthropathy and retrocalcaneal bursitis. An adventitious superficial Achilles tendon bursa may develop posterior to the Achilles tendon,[52,53] and this may be referred to as the superficial retrocalcaneal bursa[4] or retro-Achilles bursa.[54]

Many investigators have developed radiographic angles and criterion to assist in the diagnosis of Haglund syndrome. Radiographic measurements using a lateral radiograph include the Fowler-Philip angle,[55] parallel pitch lines (PPL),[56] calcaneal inclination angle,[57] and total angle.[53]

The calcaneal inclination angle is created by the intersection of a line connecting the plantar anterior tubercle and the plantar medial tuberosity with the horizontal surface. The average angle is 15 to 20°, with symptoms more likely if the angle is increased. In a series of 65 patients with Haglund syndrome, Ruch[57] found the average inclination angle of symptomatic patients to be 34°, with a range from 20 to 52°. Vega and colleagues[53] found an average inclination angle of 28° in a series of 20 symptomatic patients.

The Fowler-Philip angle (or posterior calcaneal angle) is created by the intersection of a line tangential to the posterosuperior surface of the bursal projection and greater tuberosity with another line tangential to the inferior border of the calcaneus. An angle of more than 75° was originally reported to cause symptoms.[55] Many investigators, however, have refuted that claim. Among them, Ruch,[57] Pavlov and colleagues,[56] and Lu and colleagues[46] all found that there was no statistically significant relationship between the Fowler-Phillip angle and symptoms associated with Haglund syndrome. Currently, the Fowler-Phillip angle is rarely used alone for diagnosis.

The total angle is the sum of the Fowler-Philip angle and the calcaneal inclination angle. The average total angle is between 64 and 89°,[57] with symptoms reported in those greater than 90°.

PPLs are drawn by first creating a line tangential to the inferior border of the calcaneus (also known as the calcaneal inclination line), then drawing a line perpendicular to the inclination line and connecting it with the posterior lip of the talar articular facet. The final line is made perpendicular to the second line and therefore parallel to the calcaneal inclination line, and extending posteriorly from the posterior lip of the talar articular facet towards the Achilles tendon. Normally the bursal projection should be below the superior line,[56] and portions above the line are often considered pathologic (**Fig. 6**). Pavlov and colleagues[56] found a (+) bursal projection above the PPL in 7 of 10 symptomatic patients (70%), and in only 23 of 78 control patients (30%), which was statistically significant to correlate a positive parallel pitch line with symptomatic Haglund. Among the control group, 15 of the 78 patients had clinically visible pump bumps, and each of the 15 had (+) PPL; 10 of the 15 had either isolated retrocalcaneal bursitis or Achilles tendinitis. Conversely, Lu and colleagues[46] found no statistically significant difference in parallel pitch measurements between 37 heels with Haglund symptoms (56.8% positive) versus 40 (42.5% positive) asymptomatic heels.

Retrocalcaneal exostoses can take the form of a spur of bone attached to the posterior calcaneus and projecting superiorly along the line of the Achilles tendon, or may be separate ossifications or calcifications within the soft tissue. Morris and colleagues[58]

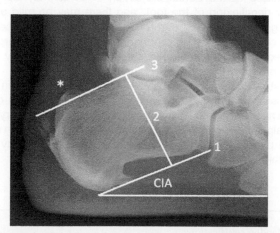

Fig. 6. Lateral radiograph of the heel showing PPL and a calcaneal inclination angle. Line 1 is a line tangential to the inferior calcaneal surface. Line 2 is perpendicular to line 1, extending to the posterior lip of the posterior facet. Line 3 is perpendicular to line 2, and thus parallel to line 1. Area above line 3, marked by asterisks, is a pathologic area. CIA, calcaneal inclination angle.

classified retrocalcaneal spurs according to their location (**Table 1**). The most common spur, classified as type 1 (**Fig. 7**), was described as a true extension of mature calcaneal bone projecting off the posterior calcaneus. Type 2 spurs were defined as separate calcifications within soft tissue 0.5 to 3 cm above the Achilles insertion (**Fig. 8**), and were often linear or ovoid. Type 3 spurs were described as calcifications within soft tissue and were found from 3 to 12 cm above the Achilles insertion.[58] These were the least common type.

The location of the spur in relation to the Achilles tendon has caused much debate, because it was traditionally thought to be intratendinous. Most investigators now consider the spur to be behind the Achilles tendon, and not wholly encompassed within it. In 1997, Chao and colleagues[59] described retrocalcaneal spur formation in cadaver specimens that were identified lateral and posterior to the Achilles tendon insertion, with no tendinous attachment on the posterior aspect of the spur (**Fig. 9**).

Multiple reasons as to why calcaneal spurring can develop over time have been theorized. In the 1930s, Ghormley[60] described that the spurs were related to posterior heel trauma and portrayed them as tendonitis ossificans traumatica, a variant of myositis ossificans. He also referred to the origin of spur ossification as periosteal. Another popular idea relates to the pull of the Achilles tendon and the chronic stressors it endures. Rufai and colleagues[61] held that this traction results in longitudinal tears and calcification. Retrocalcaneal spurring is also associated with acromegaly and seronegative arthritides.

A diagnosis for posterior heel pain should be made based on a combination of subjective complaints, clinical examination, and radiographic findings. Most patients with Haglund syndrome patients complain of dull or achy pain in the posterior heel region that is exacerbated by tight heel counters. On examination, patients may have an erythematous or hyperkeratotic posterosuperolateral prominence that is tender to palpation. When an insertional spur or enlarged insertional shelf is present, careful examination must be undertaken to assess the true cause; specifically whether the obvious retrocalcaneal spur is indeed the cause or whether the retrocalcaneal bursa and bursal projection above the insertion is to blame. Pain localized to the bursal projection or bursa may be exacerbated by plantar flexion or dorsiflexion of the foot, and there may be mild adjacent Achilles tendinitis. Radiographic markers can often help localize the point of maximal tenderness. The calcaneus may be prominent because of an enlarged or hypertrophic bursal projection, or an increased calcaneal inclination may make a normal projection more prominent.

Patients with retrocalcaneal heel exostoses often complain of pain associated with chronic strenuous activity and uphill walking. Passive dorsiflexion or active plantar flexion of the foot may recreate the symptoms, and loss of dorsiflexory range of motion may be found. Palpation along the tendon for swelling and crepitation can help localize the origin of the pain.[62] Examination of the contralateral limb may show unilateral Achilles tendon thickening on the symptomatic side.

Table 1 Type of Achilles tendon calcifications	
Type 1	Posterior calcaneus/mature bone
Type 2	0.5–3.0 cm superior to insertion/soft tissue
Type 3	Up to 12 cm proximal to insertion site/soft tissue

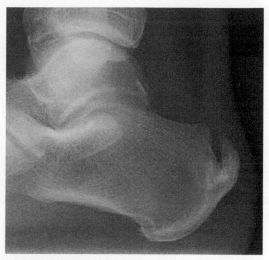

Fig. 7. Lateral radiograph. Spur extending from the posterior heel is composed of mature bone, attached to the calcaneus, and is a type 1 spur.

Cavus feet in general and specific Root Biomechanics foot types such as compensated rearfoot varus and compensated forefoot valgus have been associated with the development of Haglund syndrome.[57,63] Change in shoe gear, worn shoe gear, and sudden increase in activity or workload could also induce posterior heel pain. Haglund syndrome may affect either sex; however, women have a higher incidence.[53,55,57,64,65] It most commonly affects patients in their second and third decade of life.[56]

Differential diagnoses for painful posterior heel may include but are not limited to Achilles tendinitis,[64] retrocalcaneal exostosis,[66] infection, osteoid osteoma, diffuse

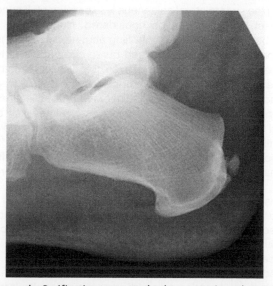

Fig. 8. Lateral radiograph. Ossification not attached to posterior calcaneus, less than 3.0 cm above insertion is a type 2 spur.

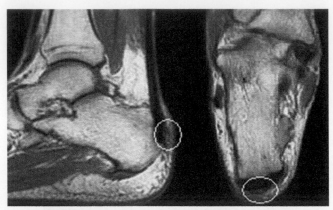

Fig. 9. Sagittal T1 MRI image on the left and transverse T1 MRI image on the right. Spur can be identified as the gray area behind the Achilles on both views.

idiopathic hyperostosis syndrome,[67] systemic inflammatory disease,[68] and lumbosacral radiculitis.

Conservative treatment is geared towards symptomatic relief and return to full function. First-line treatment may be aimed at simply reducing the pressure on the posterior heel via changing footgear or discontinuing shoes with rigid heel counters, application of horseshoe-shaped pads inside the heel counter, use of clogs, and other open-back shoes or various over-the-counter paddings available. Rest, antiinflammatory treatments, cryotherapy or ice, immobilization, and/or physical therapy can be effective at reducing symptoms. The addition of a heel lift may help by repositioning the prominence in relation to the heel counter or decreasing the tension on a symptomatic tendon, but can occasionally cause increased pain depending on the shoe itself. In anterior cavus feet, the heel lift may also help by decreasing the calcaneal inclination angle, thus making the superolateral calcaneus less prominent. If successful, orthotics incorporating a heel lift could then be considered. Nonsteroidal antiinflammatory medications have been successful in controlling acute exacerbations. Local injection of corticosteroid or aspiration of an inflamed bursa or adjacent to tendinopathy has also been documented. Caution is urged given the close proximity to the Achilles tendon. Some investigators recommend immobilization for 2 to 6 weeks after corticosteroid injection adjacent to the Achilles.[69] Theobald and colleagues[51] also advised caution in these injections, because corticosteroids are known to cause atrophy of adipose cells, and the relationship between fat in the Kager triangle and the retrocalcaneal recess continues to emerge. Recently, Sofka and colleagues[70] reported on the success of ultrasound guidance for injection directly into a painful retrocalcaneal bursa, and this may prove to be the safest modality for corticosteroid injection into the area.

Surgery is considered for those patients who fail to respond to conservative therapy after 3 to 6 months. The most commonly reported procedure for Haglund syndrome is resection of the bursal projection or posterosuperior prominence of the calcaneus, with removal of the inflamed retrocalcaneal bursa if present. Resection of a retrocalcaneal spur or calcification can be performed for those patients in which pain is directly correlated, but the senior authors has had instances in which simple bursal projection resection relieved symptoms despite large retrocalcaneal spurs evident on the radiograph (**Fig. 10**).

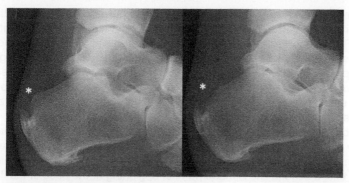

Fig. 10. Lateral radiograph, preoperatively on the left and postoperatively on the right. Patient presented with pain at the bursal projection, but with no pain in the Achilles insertion or at the retrocalcaneal spur identified on radiograph. Surgery performed to remove an inflamed bursa and the bursal projection (indicated by *asterisk*), without removing spur or detaching Achilles. Postoperatively, the patient was asymptomatic.

The only other alternative surgical technique commonly reported involves creating a dorsally based closing wedge osteotomy of the calcaneus, sometimes referred to as the Keck and Kelly osteotomy.[71]

Multiple outcomes studies for the open approach with partial resection of the posterior calcaneal tuberosity and bursectomy have shown good results.[44,72-75] Brunner and colleagues[73] reported on 39 heels with resection of the superoposterior calcaneal projection, removal of calcification in the Achilles, and use of Mitek anchor only in those heels in which the insertion of the Achilles was compromised. Of the respondents in his study, 86% stated they would repeat the procedure. The mean postoperative American Orthopaedic Foot and Ankle Society (AOFAS) score was 86, up 32 from the preoperative mean score. Chen and Huang[74] reported on 30 heels that underwent calcaneal ostectomy and found a 90% cure rate, although the eventual recovery was delayed 6 to 24 months after the procedure in 83% of the heels. Huber[75] reported on long-term outcomes of ostectomy, and found that 80 out of 98 heels were pain-free and 14 out of 98 heels had only minor discomfort after an average of 8.3 years' follow-up. Two heels in Huber's study were unchanged, and 2 were worse after the procedure. He found his long-term results directly correlated to the amount of the bursal projection removed. Those patients with complete resection of the bursal projection above the Achilles insertion via a gentle sloping osteotomy faired the best; those left with more bone above the insertion had more symptoms.

Schneider and colleagues[76] reported less favorable outcomes and found that only 69% of patients had improvement of symptoms, and 14% had worsening of symptoms after a mean follow-up of 4 years and 7 months after superoposterior calcaneus resection. Nesse and Finsen[77] reported good results in only 20 of 35 heels (57%) and satisfactory results in 10 of 35 heels (28.5%) treated with bony resection that were followed up an average of 3 years postoperatively.

Various incisions have been described, including posteromedial, posterolateral, lazy-L, transverse, J-shaped, and direct midline. Lateral incisions seem to be the most commonly reported, because vitals structures can usually be avoided. Care should be taken to avoid damaging the sural nerve or the lesser saphenous vein.[53,66] Anderson and colleagues[78] reported on a retrospective review of 31 patients who underwent a tendon-splitting approach to Haglund syndrome versus 32 patients who underwent a lateral approach. The patients in the lateral incision group reported a greater increase in AOFAS score (54- vs 43-point increase), but those in the central incision group returned to normal function at a much faster pace (4.1 months vs 6.4 months). For extensive deformity, a bilateral longitudinal incision on either side of the Achilles tendon may be used; however, this may cause the most damage to local blood supply and should also be used with caution. After soft tissue dissection and retraction of the Achilles tendon, the bursal projection is resected using an osteotome or sagittal saw, with many investigators advocating resection starting just above the Achilles insertion to avoid complications.

Sella and colleagues,[44] using a partial removal of the Achilles tendon, planned the ostectomy according to a preoperative radiographic evaluation. On a lateral radiograph, a line is drawn along the plantar aspect of the calcaneus (calcaneal inclination line). After this, a second line is made parallel beginning at the base of the flare of the anterior calcaneal process. One more line is drawn from the base of the flare of the deformity on the posterior and superior tuberosity to intersect the third line that is the most posterior point of the calcaneus. The area posterior to this line represents the cone to be removed. Using this technique, 13 of the 16 heels operated on had a good result and 3 patients had poor results.

An endoscopic decompression approach has also been described in the literature, with results statistically similar to the open technique reported.[79] The bursa may be removed using a hooded full-radius synovial shaver, and the bony deformity can be removed using a small abrader. Similar to the open technique, care must be taken to avoid the sural nerve and the calcaneal branches of the lateral plantar nerve. Aggressive resection is recommended, but removing too much bone can cause Achilles tendon avulsion or rupture.[79-81] Postoperatively, patients are placed in a non–weight-bearing cast for 1 to 2 weeks and then transitioned into walking casts for the next 2 weeks. Once the patient has returned to shoes, a 13.8-cm (5 and 7/16-inch) tapered heel lift is gradually reduced over the next 3 months.[80]

Surgical correction with complete or partial detachment and reattachment of the Achilles tendon has also been described. Sammarco and Taylor[72] reported on 34 heels and documented 17 excellent, 15 good, and 1 poor result using Maryland foot score. DeVries and Summerhays[82] reported a similar approach on 17 heels and had 16 good-to-excellent results and 1 somewhat unsatisfied patient. Complications in this study included pulmonary embolism, painful scar, transient sural neuritis, and recurrent retrocalcaneal bursitis.[82]

Various successful methods of reattachment of the Achilles have been described by investigators who have purposefully or inadvertently removed a portion of the Achilles insertion; these include deep sutures to surrounding calcaneal periosteum, use of one or more soft tissue anchors, and use of tendons transfers with interference screw for tendon augmentation, especially in instances of debridement of associated tendinosis.[72,73,83-85] Kolodziel and colleagues[86] in 1999 investigated specifically when to use augmentation or anchoring after Achilles detachment. They resected the Achilles insertion of cadaver specimens in 25% increments and then subjected the specimens to repeated cyclical loading of 3 times body weight. They found that if detachment proceeded superiorly to inferiorly, there were no avulsions with up to 50% detachment of the Achilles, and only 1 failure in 9 limbs with up to 75% detachment. Despite this result, Mafulli and colleagues[85] thought that because the cadaver testing was not done with pathologic specimens, the results could not be entirely trusted in patients with tendinopathy. They advocated the use of 2 Mitek anchors if 33% to 50% of the insertion was detached, 3 anchors if 50% to 75% was detached, 4 anchors if 75% to 99% was detached, and 5 anchors if completely detached, and reported no avulsions or loss of muscle strength in 21 cases using this protocol.[85]

In 2002, Boberg and Anania[87] described using a posterior transverse incisional approach to retrocalcaneal spurs that required minimal reflection of the Achilles tendon, followed by rongeur removal of the exostosis. Around the same time, Perez and colleagues[88] wrote about a similar transverse incisional approach with usage of an osteotome for spur removal. Both articles reported that the non–weight-bearing postoperative period was appreciably shortened, because the Achilles tendon remained intact having not been reflected to excise an extratendinous spur.

A dorsally based closing wedge osteotomy of the superior calcaneal tuberosity has been used with success to treat symptomatic Haglund syndrome as described by Keck and Kelly.[71] The osteotomy is advocated for use in patients with a high calcaneal inclination angle, enlargement of the entire posterior calcaneus,[89] and the senior author (S.V.) has had success in treating patients with recurrent or recalcitrant pain after retrocalcaneal exostectomy or bursal projection resection. The osteotomy can be fixated with the use of 1 or 2 screws, staples, or claw plates. A major benefit is that there is no need for detachment and reattachment of the Achilles; however, postoperative immobilization is needed to allow for osteotomy healing, and the calcaneal shortening inherent in the osteotomy may cause muscle weakness because of decreasing the moment arm of the Achilles tendon.[72]

AUTHORS' PREFERRED METHOD

In practice, the senior author (S.V.) commonly combines clinical examination with the calcaneal inclination angle to determine the course of treatment, and although the total angle and PPL may be drawn, he anecdotally finds them to be unreliable and falsely negative.

The senior author approaches surgical treatment after failure of conservative measures by localizing pain clinically and radiographically to the retrocalcaneal spur, the bursal projection lateral or medial to the Achilles, the Achilles itself at the level of the bursal projection or higher, or the Achilles at the insertion:

- For pain isolated to the bursal projection, regardless of results of PPL or spurring, the bursal projection is resected. If the calcaneal inclination angle is greater than 30°, a dorsally based wedge osteotomy may be added.
- For pain isolated to a retrocalcaneal spur or insertion with evidence of a spur, the spur is resected. The bursal projection is usually resected as well.
- For patients who have had recurrence after previous spur or bursal projection removal, consideration for a dorsally based wedge osteotomy is given.

To perform a simple open resection of the bursal projection without detaching the Achilles, the patient is positioned prone. A linear incision is created just lateral to the Achilles and may be flared slightly anteriorly at the distal-most aspect if additional exposure is needed. The posterosuperior aspect of the calcaneus is palpated and identified with a Freer elevator to provide a landmark, and then a deep incision is made down to the bone just lateral to the Achilles and parallel to the skin incision. The foot is plantar flexed to relax the Achilles, and the tendon is retracted superomedially. Often, rough hemorrhagic tissue is identified between the Achilles and the bursal projection, which is associated with bursitis, and this tissue is resected. The anterior surface of the Achilles is then followed distally to its insertion, and the osteotomy is initiated just above this point (**Fig. 11**). Care must be taken to visualize where the osteotomy exits superiorly on the calcaneus to avoid extending the line into or directly adjacent to the posterior facet. The cut is angled approximately 30 to 45° down from the coronal plane. The bursal projection is removed and the medial and

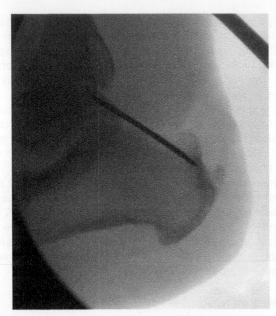

Fig. 11. Lateral intraoperative fluoroscopy. Osteotome shown within the ostectomy, confirming the amount of bone to be resected and the angle of resection. Note that it does not invade the posterior facet or the Achilles insertion, which is indicated by a ridge of bone on the posterior calcaneus.

lateral edges of the bone are smoothed with a rasp. The senior author has not found it necessary to perform preoperative calculations for the amount of bone to be resected. Patients are placed in an Ace wrap and surgical shoe, and allowed to bear weight immediately, usually without the need for formal physical therapy.

If Achilles tendon detachment cannot be avoided for complete bursal resection or if symptomatic retrocalcaneal spurs require detachment of the tendon, deep sutures from the Achilles to surrounding periosteum are used for detachments involving less than 25% of the tendon. This is augmented with 1 to 3 soft tissue anchors if it is

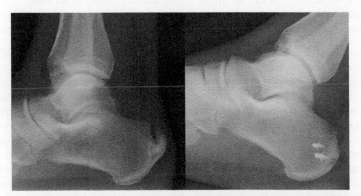

Fig. 12. Lateral preoperative radiograph on the left showing large symptomatic type 1 retrocalcaneal spur and bursal projection. Lateral postoperative radiograph on the right shows complete removal of the spur, bursal projection resection, and 2 soft tissue anchors in place for reattachment of Achilles. Postoperatively, the patient was asymptomatic.

estimated that 25% to 75% of the insertion has been detached (**Fig. 12**). Patients are then placed in a non–weight-bearing posterior splint postoperatively, with physical therapist-assisted PROM started in week 3 to 4, AROM is added in week 5, and strengthening is begun in week 6. Patients become partial weight bearing in a cast boot/walker during week 6 to 7.

SUMMARY

Thorough knowledge of normal and abnormal anatomy is key to treating painful prominences of the heel. Most posterior and plantar prominences can be successfully treated conservatively, and surgical results have been generally proved effective for patients who are recalcitrant to conservative care.

REFERENCES

1. Dunn JE, Link CL, Felson DT. Prevalence of foot and ankle conditions in a multi-ethnic community sample of older adults. Am J Epidemiol 2004;159:491–8.
2. Hill CL, Gill T, Menz H, et al. Predictors of podiatry utilisation in Australia: the North West Adelaide Health Study. J Foot Ankle Res 2008;1:8. DOI:10.1186/1757-1146-1-2.
3. Folman Y, Wosk J, Voloshin A, et al. Cyclic impacts on heel strike: a possible biomechanical factor in the etiology of degenerative disease of the human locomotor system. Arch Orthop Trauma Surg 1986;104:363–5.
4. Draves DJ. Osteology of the foot. In: Draves DJ, editor. Anatomy of the lower extremity. Baltimore (MD): Williams & Wilkins; 1986. p. 113–9.
5. Hyer CF, Dawson JM, Philbin TM, et al. The peroneal tubercle: description, classification, and relevance to peroneus longus tendon pathology. Foot Ankle Int 2005;26(11):947–50.
6. Burman M. Stenosing tendovaginitis of the foot and ankle; studies with special reference to the stenosing endovaginitis of the peroneal tendons of the peroneal tubercle. Arch Surg 1953;67:686–98.
7. Burman M. Subcutaneous tear of the tendon of the peroneus longus; its relation to the giant peroneal tubercle. Arch Surg 1956;73:216–9.
8. Trevino S, Gould N, Korson R. Surgical treatment of stenosing tenosynovitis at the ankle. Foot Ankle 1981;2:37–45.
9. Chen YJ, Hsu RW, Huang TJ. Hypertrophic peroneal tubercle with stenosing tenosynovitis: the results of surgical treatment. Changgeng Yi Xue Za Zhi 1998; 21(4):442–6.
10. Berenter JS, Goldman FD. Surgical approach for enlarged peroneal tubercles. J Am Podiatr Med Assoc 1989;79:451–4.
11. Ochoa LM, Banerjee R. Recurrent hypertrophic peroneal tubercle associated with peroneus brevis tendon tear. J Foot Ankle Surg 2007;46(5):403–8.
12. Bisceglis CF, Sirota AD, Dull DD. An unusual case of hypertrophied peroneal tubercles. J Am Podiatr Med Assoc 1983;73:481–2.
13. Bruce WD, Christofersen MR, Phillips DL. Stenosing tenosynovitis and impingement of the peroneal tendons associated with hypertrophy of the peroneal tubercle. Foot Ankle Int 1999;20(7):464–7.
14. Sobel M, Pavlov H, Geppert MJ, et al. Painful os peroneum syndrome: a spectrum of conditions responsible for plantar lateral foot pain. Foot Ankle Int 1994;15(3): 112–24.
15. Banks AS. McGlamry's comprehensive textbook of foot and ankle surgery. Philadelphia: Lippincott Williams and Wilkins; 2001.

16. Menz HB, Zammit GV, Landorf KB, et al. Plantar calcaneal spurs in older people: longitudinal traction or vertical compression? J Foot Ankle Res 2008;1:7–14.
17. Graham CE. Painful heel syndrome: rationale of treatment and diagnosis. Foot Ankle 1983;3:5.
18. Bassiouni M. Incidence of calcaneal spurs in osteo-arthrosis and rheumatoid arthritis, and in control patients. Ann Rheum Dis 1965;24:490–3.
19. Shama SS, Kominsky SJ, Lemont H. Prevelance of non-painful heel spur and its relation to postural foot position. J Am Podiatry Assoc 1983;73:122–3.
20. Riepert T, Drechsler T, Urban R, et al. [The incidence, age dependence and sex distribution of the calcaneal spur. An analysis of its x-ray morphology in 1027 patients of the central European population]. Rofo 1995;162:502–5 [in German].
21. Williams PL, Smibert JG, Cox R, et al. Imaging study of the painful heel syndrome. Foot Ankle 1987;7:345–9.
22. Banadda BM, Gono O, Vaz R, et al. Calcaneal spurs in a black African population. Foot Ankle 1992;13:352–4.
23. Prichasuk S, Subhadrabandhu T. The relationship of pes planus and calcaneal spur to plantar heel pain. Clin Orthop Relat Res 1994;306:192–6.
24. Lewin P. The foot and ankle. Philadelphia: Lea and Febiger; 1959.
25. McCarthy DJ, Gorecki GE. The anatomical basis of inferior calcaneal lesions. J Am Podiatry Assoc 1979;69:527.
26. Foreman MW, Green MA. The role of intrinsic musculature in the formation of inferior calcaneal exostoses. Clin Podiatr Med Surg 1990;7:217–23.
27. Rubin G, Witten M. Plantar calcaneal spurs. Am J Orthop 1963;5:38.
28. DuVries HL. Heel spur (calcaneal spur). Arch Surg 1957;74:536–42.
29. Hauser E. Diseases of the foot. Philadelphia: WB Saunders; 1939.
30. Hiss J. Functional foot disorders. Los Angeles (CA): University Publishing; 1949.
31. Bergmann JN. History and mechanical control of heel spur pain. Clin Podiatr Med Surg 1990;7:243–59.
32. Chang CC, Miltner LJ. Periostitis of the os calcis. J Bone Joint Surg 1934;16:355–64.
33. Kumai T, Benjamin M. Heel spur formation and the subcalcaneal enthesis of the plantar fascia. J Rheumatol 2002;29:1957–64.
34. Li J, Muehleman C. Anatomic relations of heel spur to surrounding soft tissues: greater variability than previously reported. Clin Anat 2007;20:950–5.
35. Sadat-Ali M. Plantar fasciitis/calcaneal spur among security forces personnel. Mil Med 1998;163:56–7.
36. Ozdemir H, Soyuncu Y, Ozgorgen M, et al. Effects of changes in heel fat pad thickness and elasticity on heel pain. J Am Podiatr Med Assoc 2004;94:47–52.
37. Davis PF, Severud E. Painful heel syndrome: results of non-operative treatment. Foot Ankle 1989;9:254–6.
38. Lynch DM, Goforth WP, Martin WP, et al. Conservative treatment of plantar fasciitis: a prospective study. J Am Podiatr Med Assoc 1988;88:375–80.
39. Tomczak RL, Haverstock BD. A retrospective comparison of endoscopic plantar fasciotomy to open plantar fasciotomy with heel spur resection for chronic plantar fasciitis/heel spur syndrome. J Foot Ankle Surg 1995;34:400–7.
40. Lane GD, London B. Heel spur syndrome: a retrospective report on the percutaneous plantar transverse incisional approach. J Foot Ankle Surg 2004;43:389–94.
41. Bazaz R, Ferkel RD. Results of endoscopic plantar fascia release. Foot Ankle Int 2007;28:549–56.
42. Haglund P. Beitrag zur Klinikder Achillessehne. Aschr Orthop Chir 1928;49:49 [in German].

43. Lesic A, Bumbasirevic M. Disorders of the Achilles tendon. Foot Ankle 2004;18: 63–75.
44. Sella E, Caminear D, McLarney E. Haglund's syndrome. J Foot Ankle Surg 1998; 37:110–4.
45. Reinherz RP, Smith BA, Henning KE. Understanding the pathologic Haglund's deformity. J Foot Ankle Surg 1990;29:432–5.
46. Lu CC, Cheng YM, Fu YC, et al. Angle analysis of Haglund syndrome and its relationship with osseous variations and Achilles tendon calcification. Foot Ankle Int 2007;28(2):181–5.
47. Sarrafian SK. Anatomy of the foot and ankle: descriptive, topographical, functional. Philadelphia: JB Lippincott; 1983. 249.
48. Lohrer H, Arentz S, Nauck T, et al. The Achilles tendon insertion is crescent-shaped: an in vitro anatomic investigation. Clin Orthop Relat Res 2008;466(9):2230–7.
49. Hartmann HO. The tendon sheaths and synovial bursae of the foot. Foot Ankle 1981;1:247–96.
50. Canoso JJ, Liu N, Traill MR, et al. Physiology of the retrocalcaneal bursa. Ann Rheum Dis 1988;47(11):910–2.
51. Theobald P, Bydder G, Dent C, et al. The functional anatomy of Kager's fat pad in relation to retrocalcaneal problems and other hindfoot disorders. J Anat 2006; 208(1):91–7.
52. Zadek I. An operation for the cure of achillo-bursitis. Am J Surg 1939;43:542–6.
53. Vega MR, Cavolo DJ, Green RM, et al. Haglund's deformity. J Am Podiatry Assoc 1984;74:129–35.
54. Hung EHY, Kwok WK, Tong MMP. Haglund syndrome - a characteristic cause of posterior heel pain. J HK Coll Radiol 2009;11:183–5.
55. Fowler A, Philip JF. Abnormality of the calcaneus as a cause of painful heel: its diagnosis and operative treatment. Br J Surg 1945;32:494–8.
56. Pavlov H, Heneghan M, Hersh A, et al. The Haglund syndrome: initial and differential diagnosis. Radiology 1982;144:83–8.
57. Ruch JA. Haglund's disease. J Am Podiatry Assoc 1974;64:1000–3.
58. Morris KL, Giacopelli JA, Granoff D. Classifications of radiopaque lesions of the tendo Achilles. J Foot Surg 1990;29:533.
59. Chao W, Deland JT, Bates JE, et al. Achilles tendon insertion: an in vitro anatomic study. Foot Ankle Int 1997;18(2):81–4.
60. Ghormley JW. Ossification of the tendo Achillis. J Bone Joint Surg 1938;20:153.
61. Rufai R, Ralphs JR, Benjamin M. Ultrastructure of fibrocartilages at the insertion of the rat Achilles tendon. J Anat 1996;189(1):185–91.
62. Paavola M, Kannus P, Jarvinen T, et al. Achilles tendinopathy. J Bone Joint Surg Am 2002;84:2062–76.
63. Stephens MM. Haglund's deformity and retrocalcaneal bursitis. Orthop Clin North Am 1994;25:41–6.
64. Fiamengo SA, Warren RF, Marshall JL, et al. Posterior heel pain associated with a calcaneal step and Achilles tendon calcification. Clin Orthop 1982; 167:203–11.
65. Berlin D, Coleman W, Nickamin A. Surgical approaches to Haglund's disease. J Foot Surg 1982;21:42–4.
66. Smith TF. Resection of common pedal prominence: navicular, calcaneus, and metatarsocuneiform. J Am Podiatry Assoc 1983;73:93–9.
67. Mata S, Fortin PR, Fitzcharles MA, et al. A controlled study of diffuse idiopathic skeletal hyperostosis: clinical feature and functional status. Medicine 1997;76: 104–17.

68. Resnick D, Feingold ML, Curd J, et al. Calcaneal abnormalities in articular disorders. Rheumatoid arthritis, ankylosing spondylitis, psoriatic arthritis, and Reiter syndrome. Radiology 1977;125:355–66.
69. Kennedy JC, Willis RB. The effect of local steroid injection on tendons: a biomechanical and microscopic correlative study. Am J Sports Med 1976;4:11–21.
70. Sofka CM, Adler RS, Positano R, et al. Haglund's syndrome: diagnosis and treatment using sonography. HSS J 2006;2:27–9.
71. Keck SW, Kelly JP. Bursitis of the posterior part of the heel. J Bone Joint Surg Am 1965;47:267.
72. Sammarco GJ, Taylor AL. Operative management of Haglund's deformity in the nonathlete: a retrospective study. Foot Ankle Int 1998;19:724–9.
73. Brunner J, Anderson J, O'Malley M, et al. Physician and patient based outcomes following surgical resection of Haglund's deformity. Acta Orthop Belg 2005;71:718–23.
74. Chen CH, Huang PJ. Surgical treatment for Haglund's deformity. Kaohsiung J Med Sci 2001;17(8):419–22.
75. Huber HM. Prominence of the calcaneus; late results of bone resection. J Bone Joint Surg Br 1992;74(2):315–6.
76. Schneider W, Niehus W, Knahr K. Haglund's syndrome: disappointing results following surgery: a clinical and radiographic analysis. Foot Ankle Int 2000; 21(1):26–30.
77. Nesse E, Finsen V. Poor results after resection for Haglund's heel. Analysis of 35 heels in 23 patients after 3 years. Acta Orthop Scand 1994;65(1):107–9.
78. Anderson JA, Suero E, O'Loughlin PF, et al. Surgery for retrocalcaneal bursitis: a tendon-splitting versus a lateral approach. Clin Orthop Relat Res 2008; 466(7):1678–82.
79. Leitze Z, Sella EJ, Aversa JM. Endoscopic decompression of the retrocalcaneal space. J Bone Joint Surg Am 2003;85:1488–96.
80. Frey C. Surgical advancements: arthoroscopic alternatives to open procedures: great toe, subtalar joint, Haglund's deformity, and tendoscopy. Foot Ankle Clin 2009;14:313–39.
81. Sella EJ. Disorders of the Achilles tendon and its insertion. Clin Podiatr Med Surg 2005;22(1):87–99.
82. DeVries J, Summerhays B. Surgical correction of Haglund's triad using complete detachment and reattachment of the Achilles tendon. J Foot Ankle Surg 2009; 48(4):447–51.
83. Watson D, Anderson RB, Davis WH. Comparison of results of retrocalcaneal decompression for retrocalcaneal bursitis and insertional Achilles tendinosis with calcific spur. Foot Ankle Int 2000;21:119–21.
84. Aranow MS. Posterior heel pain. Clin Podiatr Med Surg 2005;22:19–43.
85. Mafulli N, Testa V, Capasso G, et al. Calcific insertional Achilles tendinopathy reattachment with bone anchors. Am J Sports Med 2004;32(1):174–82.
86. Kolodziel P, Glisson RR, Nunley JA. Risk of avulsion of the Achilles tendon after partial excision for treatment of insertional tendonitis and Haglund's deformity: a biomechanical study. Foot Ankle Int 1999;20:433–7.
87. Boberg JS, Anania MC. Retrocalcaneal exostosis anatomy and a new surgical approach. J Am Podiatr Med Assoc 2002;92(10):537–42.
88. Perez M, Frerichs JA, Lutz KW. Modified surgical approach for retrocalcaneal exostectomy with early return to weight bearing. Clin Podiatr Med Surg 2003; 20(2):361–6.
89. Perlman MD. Enlargement of the entire posterior aspect of the calcaneus: treatment with the Keck and Kelly calcaneal osteotomy. J Foot Surg 1992;31(5):424–33.

Current Concepts and Techniques
in Foot and Ankle Surgery

Combined Distraction Osteogenesis and Papineau Technique for an Open Fracture Management of the Distal Lower Extremity

Vasilios D. Polyzois, MD, PhD[a],*, Spyridon Galanakos, MD[a],
Thomas Zgonis, DPM[b], Ioannis Papakostas, MD, PhD[c],
George Macheras, MD[a]

KEYWORDS

• Lower extremity • Arthrodesis • Ilizarov • External fixation
• Papineau technique

A plethora of surgical protocols have been described to treat open severe lower extremity fractures. These include and are not limited to early aggressive and repeated débridement of necrotic tissue, fracture stabilization with external fixation, early soft tissue coverage with local muscle flaps or free muscle transfers,[1–3] and staged skeletal reconstruction.[4–8] For bone defect reconstruction, different techniques have been described, including direct nonvascularized cancellous bone grafts,[9,10] open cancellous Papineau grafting,[11] bone transport using the Ilizarov bone-lengthening technique,[12] and vascularized bone grafts.[13,14]

Initial débridement with incomplete bone resection followed by repeated local soft tissue management was originally described by Papineau in 1973.[15–17] In this technique, serial local débridements are performed and followed by the excision of the infected bone and soft tissue defects whereas the posterior bone cortex is

---

[a] 4th Department of Orthopaedics, KAT General Hospital, 2 Nikis Street, 14561 Kifissia, Athens, Greece
[b] Division of Podiatric Medicine and Surgery, Department of Orthopaedic Surgery, The University of Texas Health Science Center at San Antonio, 7703 Floyd Curl Drive–MSC 7776, San Antonio, TX 78229, USA
[c] General Hospital of Limnos, Limnos 81400, Greece
* Corresponding author.
E-mail address: bpolyzois@yahoo.com

Clin Podiatr Med Surg 27 (2010) 463–467
doi:10.1016/j.cpm.2010.03.004
0891-8422/10/$ – see front matter © 2010 Published by Elsevier Inc.

preserved.[18–20] Topical treatments are usually consisting of frequent moist to dry dressings or advanced wound care modalities and until granulation tissue is formed in the resected bone and soft tissue defect. Additional cancellous bone grafting and delayed soft tissue closure may be necessary in some cases. Open autogenous cancellous bone grafting has been used to fill the resulting bone defect[20] after bone stabilization with a cast or an external fixation frame. Both 1-stage autogenous cancellous bone grafting of the defect and staged bone grafting procedures have also been reported and recommended.[21,22]

CASE REPORT

A 34-year-old man sustained an open distal tibial fracture after a motor vehicle accident. Radiographic examination of the open lower extremity revealed a severely comminuted fracture at distal tibia. After medical optimization, an emergent débridement and skeletal fixation of the fracture was performed within hours of the initial event. All of the nonviable soft tissue was removed and avascular bone segments were débrided. The fracture was initially stabilized with an Ilizarov external fixation device and the wound was packed with moist to dry dressings. At the second postoperative day, a repeat surgical débridement was performed in addition to a proximal tibial osteotomy through healthy bone. Intraoperative bone and soft tissue cultures revealed no bacterial growth. The second débridement resulted in a 5 × 3–cm defect of the distal tibia and a 6 × 14–cm defect of the overlying soft tissue. Two weeks postoperatively, an autogenous cancellous iliac crest bone graft was applied at the wound defect to stimulate soft tissue healing by secondary intention. Local wound care consisted of moist to dry dressings, which were performed by the patient every other day. Partial weight bearing was allowed 3 weeks after the described Papineau technique, and full weight bearing was allowed at 2 months postoperatively. The severe bone and soft tissue defect was bridged with the distraction osteogenesis procedure. The final stage of the procedure involved removal of the Ilizarov external fixation device at approximately 6 months and after his fracture consolidation. At 3 years postoperatively, the patient was completely asymptomatic and satisfied with his outcome (**Fig. 1**).

DISCUSSION

Several approaches have been described to reduce significant soft tissue and bone defects, including open[15,16,18] or closed bone grafting,[23] local or free muscle flap,[24] and closed wound irrigation with suction.[25] The Papineau technique was developed to assist with the management of difficult bony defects and posttraumatic osteomyelitis. Papineau and others have reported high rates of success in eradicating chronic bone infection and addressing significant bone deficits.[15,16,18,26,27]

A recent study by Archdeacon and Messerschmitt[28] suggested a modification of the Papineau technique by implementing a vacuum-assisted closure device in lieu of moist to dry dressing changes. This protocol included an aggressive excisional débridement of infected or necrotic bone, open cancellous bone autografting, and eradication of chronic infection with concomitant parenteral antibiotics. No major complications were noted but significant problems were observed mostly in patients with a history of smoking and diabetes mellitus, which has also been reported in the literature.[29–31]

In addition, recent literature has advocated the concept of internal pedal amputation in diabetic patients with multiple foot bony segmental osteomyelitis. According to the investigator, this method of pedal amputation consists of resection of the metatarsals,

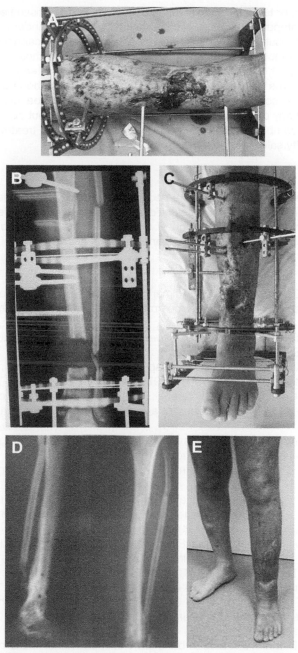

Fig. 1. Clinical picture of the lower extremity and initial application of the Ilizarov apparatus (*A*) followed by a proximal tibial osteotomy (*B*) and modified Ilizarov external fixation device and Papineau technique (*C*). Note the wound healthy margins at 2 months postoperatively. Final radiographic (*D*) and clinical pictures (*E*) at 3 years postoperatively.

midtarsal bones, or talus with preservation of the toes and soft tissue envelope. After internal pedal amputations of a diabetic patient, the foot undergoes significant contracture that results in a stable, functional, and residual limb capable of being protected in custom-molded shoe gear with external or in-shoe orthoses.[32]

In this case report, a combination of an Ilizarov distraction osteogenesis and Papineau technique was used to achieve closure of a very large bone and soft tissue defect. Extensive soft tissue and bone débridement might be necessary in the management of any open lower-extremity fracture with or without concomitant osteomyelitis. This combined technique has showed a successful treatment option for a lower-extremity salvage procedure.

SUMMARY

Staged reconstructive procedures are necessary to obtain a desirable result in any open lower-extremity fracture with significant soft tissue and bone defect. Surgical experience with an astute knowledge of external fixation use is also required and maximized through a multidisciplinary team approach effort.

REFERENCES

1. Cierny G, Byrd HS, Jones RE. Primary versus delayed soft tissue coverage for severe open tibial fractures: a comparison for results. Clin Orthop 1983;178: 54–63.
2. Green TL, Beatty ME. Soft tissue coverage for lower extremity trauma. J Orthop Trauma 1988;2(2):158–73.
3. Kojima T, Kohono T, Eto T. Muscle flap wit simultaneous mesh skin graft for skin defects of the lower leg. J Trauma 1979;19(10):724–9.
4. Behrens F, Comfort TH, Searls K, et al. Unilateral external fixation for severe open tibial fractures: preliminary report of a prospective study. Clin Orthop 1983;178: 111–20.
5. Blick SS, Brumback RJ, Lakatos R, et al. Early prophylactic bone grafting of high energy tibial fractures. Clin Orthop 1989;240:21–41.
6. Brown PW. The prevention of infection in open wounds. Clin Orthop 1973;96: 42–50.
7. Naique SB, Pearse M, Nanchahal J. Management of severe open tibial fractures: the need for combined orthopaedic and plastic surgical treatment in specialist centres. J Bone Joint Surg Br 2006;88(3):351–7.
8. Court-Brown CM, Wheelwright EF, Christie J, et al. External fixation for type III open tibial fractures. J Bone Joint Surg Br 1990;72(5):801–4.
9. Chan KM, Leung YK, Cheng JC, et al. The management of type III open tibial fractures. Injury 1984;16(3):157–65.
10. Christian ET, Bosse MJ, Robb G. Reconstruction of large diaphyseal defects without free fibular transfer in grade IIIB tibial fractures. J Bone Joint Surg Am 1989;71(7):994–1004.
11. Green SA, Diabal TA. The open bone graft for septic nonunion. Clin Orthop 1983; 180:117–24.
12. Dagher F, Roukoz S. Compound tibial fractures with bone loss treated by the Ilizarov technique. J Bone Joint Surg Br 1991;73(2):316–21.
13. Minami A, Kasashima T, Iwasaki N, et al. Vascularised fibular grafts: an experience of 102 patients. J Bone Joint Surg Br 2000;82(7):1022–5.
14. Brown KL. Limb reconstruction with vascularized fibular grafts after bone tumor resection. Clin Orthop 1991;262:64–73.

15. Papineau LJ. L'excision-greffe avec fermeture retardee deliberee dans l'osteo-myelite chronique. Nouv Presse Med 1973;2:2753–5.
16. Papineau L, Alfageme A, Dalcourt J, et al. Osteomylite chronique: excision et greffe de spongieuz a lair libre apres mises a plat extensives. Int Orthop 1979; 3:165 SICOT [in French].
17. Saleh M, Kreibich N, Ribbans WJ. Circular frames in the management of infected tibial non-union: a modification of the Papineau technique. Injury 1996;27:31–3.
18. Panda M, Ntungila N, Kalunda M, et al. Treatment of chronic osteomyelitis using the Papineau technique. Int Orthop 1998;22:37–40.
19. Mosher CM. The Papineau bone graft: a limb salvage technique. Orthop Nurs 1991;10:27–32.
20. Cabanela ME. Open cancellous bone grafting of infected bone defects. Orthop Clin North Am 1984;15:427–40.
21. Patzakis MJ, Scilaris TA, Chon J, et al. Results of bone grafting for infected tibial nonunion. Clin Orthop 1995;315:192–8.
22. Lei H, Yi L. One stage open cancellous bone grafting of infected fracture and non-union. J Orthop Sci 1998;3:318–23.
23. Oliveria JC. Bone graft and chronic osteomyelitis. J Bone Joint Surg Br 1971;53: 672–83.
24. McNally MA, Small JO, Tofighi HG, et al. Two-stage management of chronic oste-omyelitis of the long bones: the Belfast technique. J Bone Joint Surg Br 1993;75: 375–80.
25. Clawson DK, Davis FJ, Hansen ST Jr. Treatment of chronic osteomyelitis with emphasis on closed suction-irrigation technic. Clin Orthop 1973;96:88–97.
26. Tulner SA, Schaap GR, Strackee SD, et al. Long-term results of multiple stage treatment for posttraumatic osteomyelitis of the tibia. J Trauma 2004;56:633–42.
27. Emami A, Mjoberg B, Larsson S. Infected tibial nonunion. Good results after open cancellous bone grafting in 37 cases. Acta Orthop Scand 1995;66:447–51.
28. Archdeacon MT, Messerschmitt P. Modern Papineau technique with vacuum-as-sisted closure. J Orthop Trauma 2006;20:134–7.
29. Kelly PJ, Fitzgerald RH Jr, Cabanela ME, et al. Results of treatment of tibial and femoral osteomyelitis in adults. Clin Orthop 1990;259:295–303.
30. Marsh DR, Shah S, Elliott J, et al. The ilizarov method in nonunion, malunion, and infection of fractures. J Bone Joint Surg Br 1997;79:273–9.
31. Siegel HJ, Patzakis MJ, Holtom PD, et al. Limb salvage for chronictibial osteomy-elitis: an outcome study. J Trauma 2000;48:484–9.
32. Koller A. Internal pedal amputations. Clin Podiatr Med Surg 2008;25(4):641–53.

Recurrent Acute Compartment Syndrome of the Foot Following a Calcaneal Fracture Repair

Crystal L. Ramanujam, DPM, Justin Wade, DPM, Brian Selbst, DPM,
Ronald Belczyk, DPM, Thomas Zgonis, DPM*

KEYWORDS

• Calcaneal fractures • Compartment syndrome • Foot
• Fasciotomy • Trauma

Acute compartment syndrome after a sustained calcaneal fracture has been reported to occur in approximately 10% of calcaneal fracture pathology.[1] The condition is commonly associated with high-energy, crushing-type injuries, yet it can also be seen in lower-impact trauma.[2] Diagnosis can be difficult in the midst of severe pain and edema associated with the fracture itself. A high index of suspicion based on the history of injury and clinical examination usually elucidates an accurate diagnosis. Expeditious confirmation can be made with the use of a portable intracompartmental pressure monitoring device, particularly in determining the calcaneal compartment pressure.[3] Timely recognition and immediate fasciotomies are necessary for prevention of debilitating sequelae, such as tissue necrosis, joint contractures, functional impairment, and irreversible neuromuscular injury.[1,2] Few reports exist on recurrent acute compartment syndrome in the lower extremity after fasciotomies. Kotak and Bendall[4] and Hanypsiak and colleagues[5] each reported a case of recurrent acute compartment syndrome of the leg 1 year after initial fasciotomies. Batra and colleagues[6] reported a case of recurrent acute compartment syndrome after a calcaneal fracture in a patient 7 years after undergoing fasciotomies of the foot. Most of these previously published cases occurred after a second traumatic event. In contrast, this article describes a rare case demonstrating a recurrence of acute compartment syndrome within days of initial fasciotomies and surgical repair of a calcaneal fracture. In light of this case report, recurrent acute compartment syndrome of the foot cannot

Division of Podiatric Medicine and Surgery, Department of Orthopaedic Surgery, The University of Texas Health Science Center at San Antonio, 7703 Floyd Curl Drive–MSC 7776, San Antonio, TX 78229, USA
* Corresponding author.
E-mail address: zgonis@uthscsa.edu

Clin Podiatr Med Surg 27 (2010) 469–474
doi:10.1016/j.cpm.2010.03.005
0891-8422/10/$ – see front matter © 2010 Elsevier Inc. All rights reserved.

be excluded in the differential diagnosis of a patient who exhibits symptoms even after initial fascial decompression.

CASE REPORT

A previously healthy 31-year-old man presented to the authors' institution's emergency department for exponentially increasing pain to the left foot due to an injury sustained the previous day when he had tripped down a flight of stairs. The patient had jumped several steps and landed with all of his weight concentrated to the left heel. He was unable to bear weight on the affected limb and he sought immediate medical attention at an urgent care facility before his visit.

The patient denied having past surgeries and reported no history of smoking, alcohol, or drug use. Physical examination revealed the patient in no apparent distress with stable vital signs. Cardiovascular and pulmonary examinations were unremarkable and the primary musculoskeletal survey was significant only for the left lower extremity. The foot exhibited an abrasion to the hallux, edema encompassing the hindfoot and midfoot, and ecchymosis at the plantar lateral heel. Pedal pulses were nonpalpable but biphasic waveforms to the dorsalis pedis and posterior tibial arteries were audible with a Doppler ultrasound. The digits were cool to touch with slight pallor appearance when compared with the contralateral foot; however, light touch sensation was intact to the digits via 5.07-g Semmes-Weinstein monofilament. Pain was elicited on passive extension and flexion of the digits. Radiographic images of the left foot and ankle revealed an intra-articular calcaneal fracture with subtalar joint depression and varus malalignment. Due to the nature of the injury and clinical findings, compartmental pressures of the foot were immediately obtained using a portable intracompartmental pressure-monitoring device in the emergency department. The calcaneal compartment pressure measured 162 mm Hg. Informed consent was obtained from the patient for emergent fasciotomies of the foot. He was taken to the operating room 2 hours after presentation. With the patient under general anesthesia, pressures were measured again showing calcaneal compartment pressure of 120 mm Hg and 89 mm Hg in the second intermetatarsal interspace. A triple-incision fascial decompression was performed at the medial midfoot and second and fourth dorsal intermetatarsal interspaces. Large amounts of hematoma were evacuated from the incision sites. The wounds were packed open with light dressing at the initial surgery and a well-padded posterior splint was applied to the lower extremity for stability.

Three days later, once the patient's pain and edema had subsided and there was return of palpable pedal pulses, it was decided to perform an open reduction with internal fixation of the calcaneal fracture using a lateral calcaneal plate, subtalar joint fusion with 2-screw fixation, and delayed primary closure of the fasciotomy wounds. After this procedure, the limb was dressed in a well-padded posterior splint and monitored postoperatively with intravenous pain medication and prophylactic antibiotics. Within 48 hours, the patient developed a fever of 101.9°F and an elevated white blood cell count of 18,300. He admitted to severe pain in the left foot that was uncontrolled by oral or intravenous analgesics. On removal of the dressings and splint, the left foot was pale with clear fluid-filled bullae located at the lateral heel and edema and purpura from the dorsum of the foot extending to the knee. Due to the fever and elevated white blood cell count, appropriate testing to determine the source, including urinalysis, blood cultures, and chest radiograph, were completed, yet all were negative. Ultrasound of the left lower extremity was also negative for deep venous thrombosis. The patient was diagnosed with a rapid recurrence of acute compartment syndrome to the left foot and a second series of fasciotomies were performed emergently through the previous fasciotomy incisions. Postoperatively there was immediate resolution of all symptoms. The secondary fasciotomy wounds were left open for 10 days and a negative pressure wound therapy (NPWT) device was applied surgically to the wounds to allow for secondary intention healing. The patient remained stable throughout his hospital stay.

The patient completed a total of 6 weeks of outpatient NPWT with hyperbaric oxygen treatments, after which the fasciotomy wounds (medial and fourth inerspace) were closed via split thickness skin grafting. At 6 months postoperatively, the patient returned to full weight-bearing activity with radiographic evidence of fusion at the subtalar joint and union of the calcaneal fracture. The patient was last seen at the authors' clinic at 13 months after the initial injury, doing well in his daily activities with full return to work without residual foot deformity (**Fig. 1**).

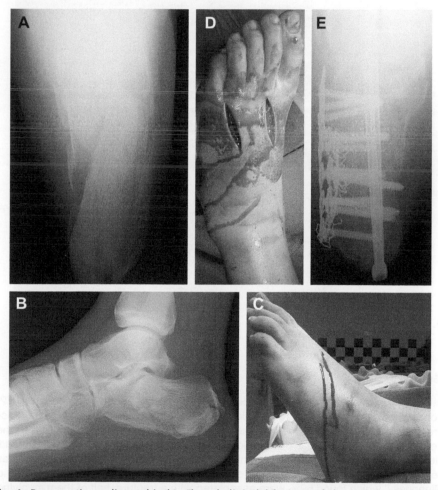

Fig. 1. Preoperative radiographic (*A, B*) and clinical (*C*) views of the initial comminuted calcaneal fracture with the acute compartment syndrome followed by foot fasciotomies (*D*). Postoperative initial radiographs (*E, F*) that were followed by a repeated and more extensive fasciotomies and NPWT application at the large medial and dorsolateral surgical wounds (*G*). Final radiographic (*H*) and clinical (*I, J*) views at 13 months' follow-up.

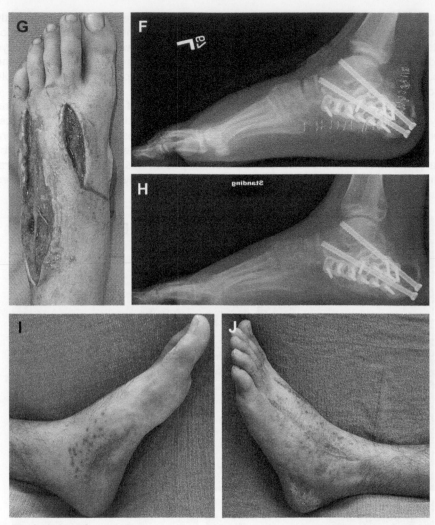

Fig. 1. (*continued*)

DISCUSSION

Acute compartment syndrome, first described by Richard vonVolkmann[7] in 1872, occurs when perfusion pressure in a closed anatomic space falls below tissue pressure. If left untreated, the condition leads to tissue necrosis, loss of function in the affected limb, neurovascular dysfunction, contractures, and, in severe cases, renal failure and death.[8] Most cases are linked directly to trauma or crushing injury as seen in a study of 164 diagnosed compartment syndromes by McQueen and colleagues,[9] which found 69% were associated with a fracture, half of them involving the tibia. The complex anatomy of the foot, composed of 9 distinct compartments (medial, lateral, superficial, calcaneal, adductor, and 4 interosseous) can make the diagnosis of acute compartment syndrome especially difficult and may be missed, thereby leading to detrimental effects.[10] Pain is the most consistent feature found in acute compartment syndrome and, although helpful for identification, the symptoms of edema, paresthesias, and neurovascular deficits are not diagnostic.[1]

Compartment syndrome directly after an acute calcaneal fracture is not uncommon; however, a recurrent acute compartment syndrome within a short time after surgical decompression of the fascial spaces is rare. In patients who have required fascial decompression, definitive repair of the calcaneal fracture is usually recommended only after the fasciotomy wounds have closed in delayed fashion.[1] In this case, once the involved limb appeared stable after the initial fasciotomies and careful postoperative monitoring, it was decided to perform open repair of the calcaneal fracture with internal fixation and delayed primary closure because the patient had severe malalignment and articular compromise.[11] Sudden onset of severe pain unrelieved by pain medication, pale appearance of the foot, and nonpitting edema after definitive fixation of the fracture led to a high index of suspicion for another episode of acute compartment syndrome. Fever and leukocytosis as seen in this patient is not diagnostic for compartment syndrome, yet other causes for these findings, such as acute infection, had been ruled out with further diagnostic testing. Use of a portable intracompartmental pressure monitoring device provides an efficient, reliable method to confirm the presence of elevated compartmental pressures.[12] Although other technologies, including near infrared spectrometry, MRI, scintigraphy, and laser Doppler flowmetry, have been reported helpful in diagnosis, these methods are nonspecific and the time required to perform them would most likely delay appropriate treatment.[13] Matsen and colleagues[14] found necrosis after 6 hours of ischemia, which currently is the accepted upper limit of viability.

Surgeons should be careful not to confuse a recurrent acute compartment syndrome with the clinically distinct condition of chronic compartment syndrome. Chronic compartment syndrome is induced by exercise or exertion causing recurrent pain and disability, usually in the legs; it subsides with cessation of the inciting activity but recurs once the activity is resumed.[15] To the authors' knowledge, previously published reports of recurrent acute compartment syndrome within days or weeks of an initial fasciotomy have been limited to the hand or forearm.[16,17] For the few cases reported in the literature regarding the lower extremity, a minimum of 1 year and up to 7 years had passed since the first fasciotomy; furthermore, the authors of those case reports were able to pinpoint a direct traumatic event leading to the second compartment syndrome.[2–4] Treatments involved repeat fasciotomies through previous incisions and delayed closure of the skin.

The recurrence of acute compartment syndrome in this case report was possibly attributable to the initial complex injury with severe hematoma and edema, possible early closure of the initial fasciotomy sites, and possible early definitive repair of the severely comminuted calcaneal fracture. Further trauma to the tissues induced by surgical manipulation can lead to hematoma formation thereby increasing pressure within the fascial spaces of the foot. Continued bleeding from the cancellous bone of the calcaneus would also contribute to elevated compartment pressures. Additionally, external pressure from postoperative compressive dressings, splints, and casts have been shown to increase the risk of compartment syndrome.[18] Further complications in this patient were avoided through immediate recognition of the condition, repeat fasciotomies, and allowing the very large wounds to heal by secondary intention through the adjunctive therapies of NPWT and hyperbaric oxygen with later skin grafting. In conclusion, this case underscores the need for surgeons to be aware of the possibility of recurrent compartment syndrome in managing traumatic foot injuries. Immediate diagnosis and appropriate treatment of a recurrent acute compartment syndrome can lead to a successful, functional outcome.

REFERENCES

1. Myerson M, Manoli A. Compartment syndromes of the foot after calcaneal fractures. Clin Orthop Relat Res 1993;290:142–50.
2. Goldman FD, Dayton PD, Hanson CJ. Compartment syndrome of the foot. J Foot Surg 1990;29:37.
3. Whitesides TE Jr, Haney TC, Harada H, et al. A simple method for tissue pressure determination. Arch Surg 1975;110:1311–3.
4. Kotak BP, Bendall SP. Recurrent acute compartment syndrome. Injury 2000;31: 66–7.
5. Hanypsiak B, Bergfeld JA, Miniaci A, et al. Recurrent compartment syndrome after fracture of a tibiofibular synostosis in a National Football League player. Am J Sports Med 2007;35:127–30.
6. Batra S, McMurtrie A, Sinha AK, et al. Recurrent compartment syndrome of foot following a calcaneal fracture. J Emerg Med 2007;13:154–6.
7. vonVolkmann R. Ischaemic muscle paralyses and contractures. 1881. Clin Orthop Relat Res 2007;456:20–1.
8. Weinmann M. Compartment syndrome. Emerg Med Serv 2003;32:36.
9. McQueen MM, Gaston P, Court-Brown CM. Acute compartment syndrome. Who is at risk? J Bone Joint Surg Br 2000;82:200–3.
10. Manoli A 2nd, Weber TG. Fasciotomy of the foot: an anatomical study with special reference to release of the calcaneal compartment. Foot Ankle 1990;10:267–75.
11. Stapleton JJ, Belczyk R, Zgonis T. Surgical treatment of calcaneal fracture malunions and posttraumatic deformities. Clin Podiatr Med Surg 2009;26:79–90.
12. Whitesides TE Jr, Haney TC, Morimoto K, et al. Tissue pressure measurements as a determinant for the need of fasciotomy. Clin Orthop 1975;113:43–51.
13. Elliott KG, Johnstone AJ. Diagnosing acute compartment syndrome. J Bone Joint Surg Br 2003;85:625–32.
14. Matsen FA, Winquist RA, Krugmire RB. Diagnosis and management of compartmental syndromes. J Bone Joint Surg Am 1980;62:286–91.
15. Pedowitz RA, Hargens AR, Mubarak SJ, et al. Modified criteria for the objective diagnosis of chronic compartment syndrome of the leg. Am J Sports Med 1990;18:35–40.
16. Kim KC, Rhee KJ, Shin HD. Recurrent dorsal compartment syndrome of the upper arm after blunt trauma. J Trauma 2008;65:1543–6.
17. Chokshi BV, Lee S, Wolfe SW. Recurrent compartment syndrome of the hand: a case report. J Hand Surg Am 1998;23(1):66–9.
18. Halanski M, Noonan KJ. Cast and splint immobilization: complications. J Am Acad Orthop Surg 2008;16:30–40.

Index

Note: Page numbers of article titles are in **boldface** type.

A

Abductor digiti minimi flap, for calcanectomy coverage, 425
Abductor hallucis flap, for calcanectomy coverage, 425
Abscess, postoperative, 395–396
Achilles tendon
  erosion of, in Reiter syndrome, 436
  insertional tendinitis of (retrocalcaneal exostosis), 450–459
  stretching of, for plantar fasciitis, 375–376
  surgery on, for retrocalcaneal exostosis, 456
  tendonitis of, 434
  tightening of, plantar fasciitis in, 371
Amputation, for osteomyelitis, 425–426
Ankylosing spondylitis, 371–372, 433–435
Anteater sign, in anterior process enlargement, 445
Antibiotics
  for foreign body, 359–360
  for osteomyelitis, 422–424, 427
Antiinflammatory agents, for plantar fasciitis, 376
Apophysitis, calcaneal, 356–358
Arthritis
  gouty, 439
  in inflammatory bowel disease, 436
  in Reiter syndrome, 372, 435–436
  in sarcoidosis, 436–437
  laboratory studies for, 432
  psoriatic, 435
  rheumatoid, 371, 432–433
Arthrodesis, overcorrection or undercorrection in, 397–399
Arthropathy, Charcot, after calcaneal surgery, 403
Athletes foot, 413
Atrophy, dermal, 411–412
Auspitz sign, in psoriatic arthritis, 435

B

Basal cell carcinoma, 413–414
Biopsy, bone, for osteomyelitis, 420
Blisters, friction, 412
Bone
  biopsy of, for osteomyelitis, 420
  contusion of, 373
  infections of. *See* Osteomyelitis.

Clin Podiatr Med Surg 27 (2010) 475–484
doi:10.1016/S0891-8422(10)00054-6
0891-8422/10/$ – see front matter ∠ 2010 Elsevier Inc. All rights reserved.

podiatric.theclinics.com

Moving?

Make sure your subscription moves with you!

To notify us of your new address, find your **Clinics Account Number** (located on your mailing label above your name), and contact customer service at:

Email: journalscustomerservice-usa@elsevier.com

800-654-2452 (subscribers in the U.S. & Canada)
314-447-8871 (subscribers outside of the U.S. & Canada)

Fax number: 314-447-8029

Elsevier Health Sciences Division
Subscription Customer Service
3251 Riverport Lane
Maryland Heights, MO 63043

Printed and bound by CPI Group (UK) Ltd, Croydon, CR0 4YY

03/10/2024

01040447-0013